HOME MADE NATURAL REMEDIES AND ESSENTIAL OILS

Effective ways to get Rid of Mucus and Phlegms with Natural Remedies & Essential Oils

BONUS! INCLUDING NATURAL REMEDIES TO RELIEVE COLD AND FLU FOR CHILDREN & TODDLERS

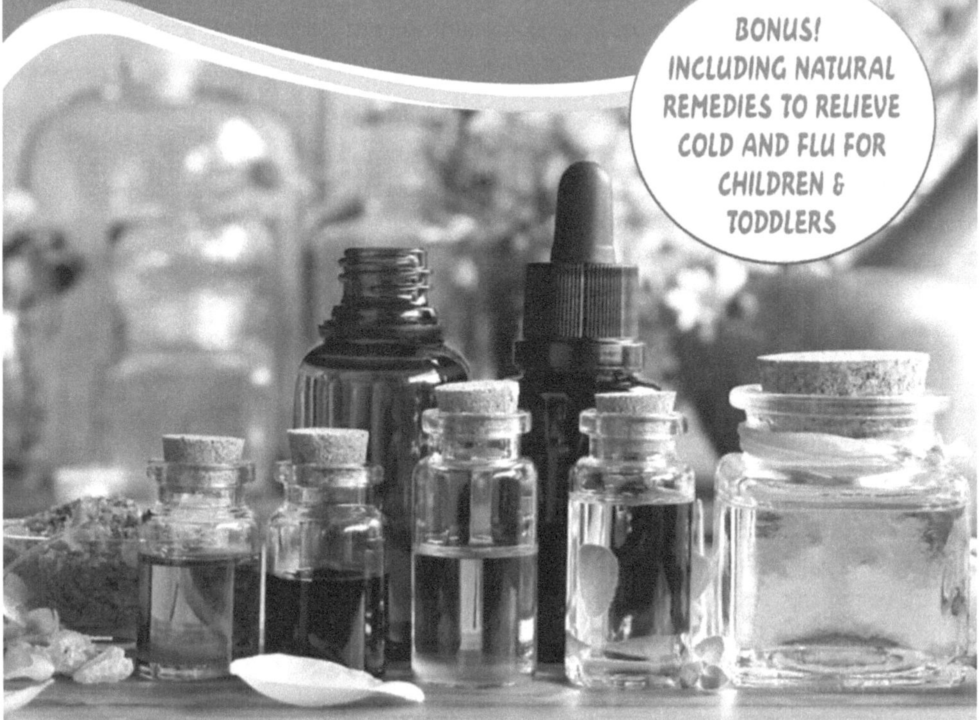

ANNE-MARIE COLLINGWOOD & ERICK WILTSHIRE

© Copyright 2019 by Anne-Marie Collingwood & Erick Wiltshire

All rights reserved.

This document is geared towards providing exact and reliable information with regard to the topic and issue covered. The publication is sold with the idea that the publisher is not required to render accounting, officially permitted, or otherwise, qualified services. If advice is necessary, legal or professional, a practiced individual in the profession should be ordered.

- From a Declaration of Principles which was accepted and approved e□ually by a Committee of the American Bar Association and a Committee of Publishers and Associations.

In no way is it legal to reproduce, duplicate, or transmit any part of this document in either electronic means or in printed format. Recording of this publication is strictly prohibited and any storage of this document is not allowed unless with written permission from the publisher. All rights reserved.

The information provided herein is stated to be truthful and consistent, in that any liability, in terms of inattention or otherwise, by any usage or abuse of any policies, processes, or directions contained within is the solitary and utter responsibility of the recipient reader. Under no circumstances will any legal responsibility or blame be held against the publisher for any reparation, damages, or monetary loss due to the information herein, either directly or indirectly.

Respective authors own all copyrights not held by the publisher.

The information herein is offered for informational purposes solely and is universal as so. The presentation of the information is without contract or any type of guarantee assurance.

The trademarks that are used are without any consent, and the publication of the trademark is without permission or backing by the trademark owner. All trademarks and brands within this book are for clarifying purposes only and are owned by the owners themselves, not affiliated with this document.

TABLE OF CONTENTS

INTRODUCTION

CONCLUSION

INTRODUCTION

In today's world, lifestyle patterns and trends are in constant flux. They come and go before we know it. But one of the modern trends which are here to stay is the use of natural remedies. And we should be very grateful for it.

Natural remedies can be used for a plethora of ailments, big or small, and it can be made very easily at home just by using natural components such as vegetables, fruits, and herbs. And some of the many advantages that using natural remedies offers are that it is simple and yet cost-effective, has no side effects or does not contain harmful chemicals and it also gives you the chance to be your very own doctor!

The best way to start using natural remedies to your advantage is from your own kitchen. You will find a cure for almost every other problem: from a common cold to your teenager's acne issues to your mother in-law's knee aches. Once you have mastered some cures and methods, you can try using more difficult to find herbs and natural products. You can use natural remedies, not just to cure ailments, but also to stay healthy in general and avoid small, day to day diseases. Using natural medication will also help you to build up your immune system extraordinarily. Although, we suggest you read up thoroughly before starting any application of remedies and you will be able to help anyone: from your toddler to your grandma.

Natural remedies, unlike antibiotics, do not stuff you up with excessive chemicals; instead they help you to achieve well being with the use of chemicals that are naturally present in the vegetables, fruits, and any herbs. Using antibiotics can have a lot of bad effects such as weakness, allergies, excessive drowsiness, and diarrhea.

In ancient times, people were very practical and they knew how to make the most of the resources that were available to them. They even used as much knowledge as was available from various other places. A plethora of information on herbal formulas was available from Indians. Over the ages, a lot has been discovered about the human body and nutrition which has helped in accurately pointing out diseases in specific body parts and their cures. We should make the best use of this knowledge and reinforce research and development in this field.

Through regular and accurate use of natural remedies, you can treat more than 500 disorders and diseases. You will find a cure to everyday illnesses such as acne, acidity, body pains, toothache, colds, back pain, hair loss, headache, weight loss, eye's vision, and even wounds. You can even strengthen your immune system and prevent hair loss, acne, dandruff, aches, cuts, and burns. Natural remedies are possibly the best therapy to cure infections that too without any side effects.

In this eBook, you will discover Home Made Natural Remedies and Essential Oils and their uses as well as their effective ways to get rid of phlegm and mucus.

REASONS WHY HOME REMEDIES ARE SO BENEFICIAL

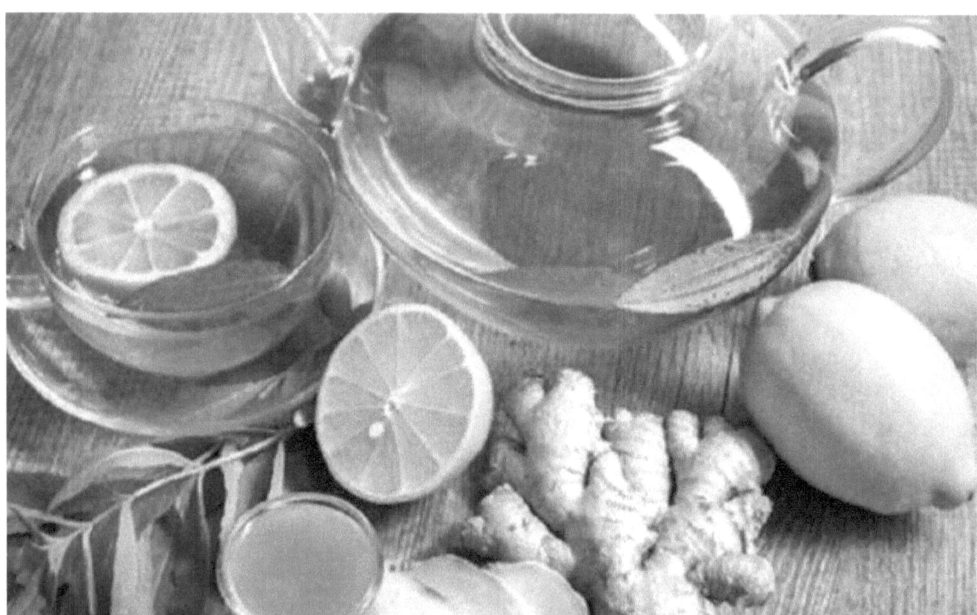

The usage of home remedies to treat any type of disease is not supernatural. Vegetables and fruits and even spices and herbs have been widely recommended to cure various illnesses. They were also used earlier as forms of medications. The old generation used this kind of treatment for quite some time until modern medicine took over. Many however still prefer the old style of treating diseases in their daily lives as they have been widely proven to be more beneficial than their counterparts that are served over the counter.

Benefits of Home Remedies

- ❖ **Cheap:** Drugs made by big pharmaceutical companies are very costly as they undergo processing, advertisement, and marketing just like a commercial commodity. Herbal remedies, on the other hand, are cheaper to make.
- ❖ **Clean:** As raw materials for natural remedies are the same ingredients employed in cooking, cleanliness is assured. When you compare them to other commercial medicinal products, preparation is more assuring.
- ❖ **Easy to find:** Because natural methods need only spices, vegetables, herbs, and fruits, getting the right one for any kind of mild illnesses is not difficult. In the past, when several people grew various plants in the backyard, there was a strong likelihood of getting medicinal plants. Similarly today, because more

people are increasingly living in urban areas, spices, fruits, medicinal plants, and vegetables are available in area supermarkets. Just look for apple, garlic, honey, ginger, lemon, thyme, celery and other vegetables and fruits that can offer a variety of medicinal benefits.

❖ **Milder**: Unlike most over-the-counter medicines and syrups, natural medicine is unspoiled and of course fresh. The contents of such medicine are very pure and attack the disease that you intend to cure directly. Because it is natural, it has no strong components as compared to over-the-counter medications.

❖ **More effective:** Homeopathic remedies cure a variety of mild diseases. Simple honey, garlic, or ginger may treat various kinds of mild diseases. They may cure acidity, pimples, age spots, athlete foot, abdomen pain, heartburn, acne scars, arthritis, backache, baldness, bad breath, bites and stings, fat belly, blood pressure, bleeding gums, bronchitis, bruises, sinus, burns, cold sores, canker sores, constipation, common cold, cuts, leg cramps, dandruff, depression, diarrhea, ear infection, fat thighs, flu, swimmer's ear, eczema, fat hips, food poisoning, yeast infection, gingivitis, worms, gout, water retention, hemorrhoids, toothache, heart exhaustion, tired eyes, piles, sunburns, hiccups, stretch marks, head lice, sore throats, indigestion, snoring, low blood skin allergies, sugar, sensitive teeth, migraine, ringworms, headache, rheumatism, weak memory, pimples, mouth ulcers, obesity, nausea, hemorrhoids or piles peptic ulcers among many others.

❖ **Few side effects:** Medications served over the counter have various ingredients that attack the intended illnesses, but this does not stop here. However, these medications are associated with a number of side effects that affect other body functions. The most common one being drowsiness. On the other hand, side effects are minimal when herbal remedies are used as they only target pure medicinal functions.

HOME MADE REMEDIES FOR DIABETES

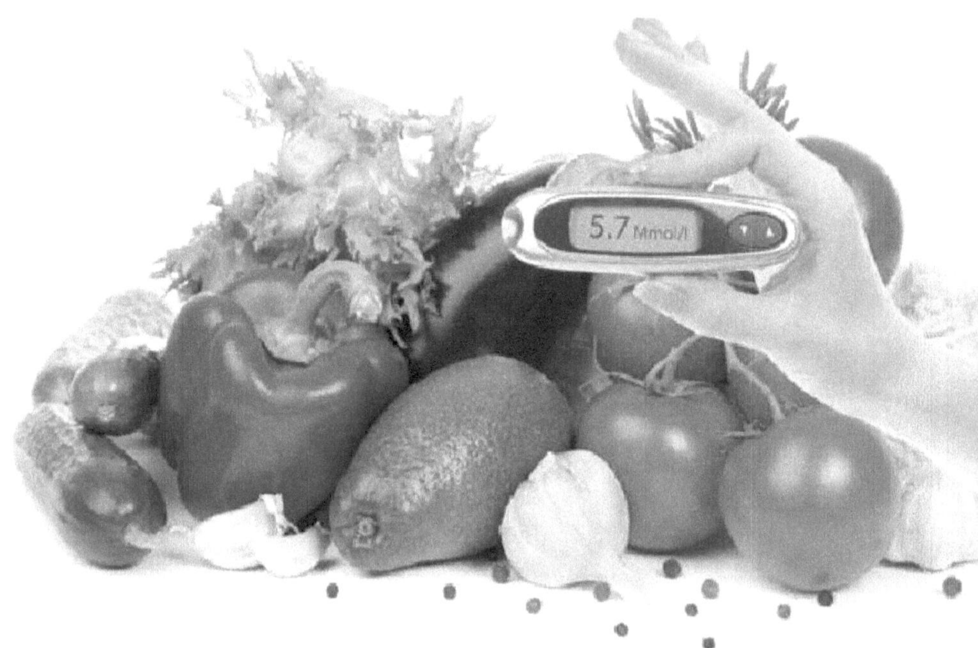

The metabolic disorder that hinders the utilization of glucose completely and partially is known as diabetes. Diabetes can further be of two types namely: 1-diabetes Mellitus (insulin-dependent diabetes) and 2-diabetes Mellitus (non-insulin-dependent diabetes). In 1 type of diabetes, the blood sugar level is not normal due to the inefficiency of the body to produce sufficient insulin and in type number 2, the cells are unable to respond properly to the insulin. The first type of diabetes generally occurs during childhood or adolescence but other ages are also attacked. In order to be healthy these patients need insulin daily. The normal blood sugar without having food is between 80 to 120 mg/dl and this can move up a level of 160mg/dl within two hours after having your meals. The second type of diabetes is found mostly in adults and specifically in those who are overweight and over forty years old. These people can control the sugar level in their blood by controlling their weight along with regular exercise and a balanced diet.

Some of the basic symptoms of diabetes are increased thrust, urination very frequently, an appetite increase, able to feel weakness and loss of weight along with erection problems. The probable causes of diabetes are insulin deficiency or resistance, high blood pressure, high cholesterol, a life full of stress and burdens and eating excessively. It is also a hereditary disease and can be transferred to you by your parents.

Some homemade natural remedies for curing diabetes in an effective manner are as follows:

1. In one glass of water, you need to boil fifteen fresh leaves of mango and leave it for one night. In the morning filter this and drink it. This should be the first thing you need to intake in the morning.
2. Half teaspoon of ground day leaf and half teaspoon of turmeric needs to be mixed with one tablespoon of gel of Aloe Vera. The mixture should be taken twice a day before lunch and dinner.
3. Small Bitter Gourd's watery juice with its seed removed should be drunk two times every day. This is considered to be the best natural remedy for diabetes.
4. In one liter of boiling water add 3- tablespoons of cinnamon and simmer it for the duration of twenty minutes in a low flame. Now strain the mixture and drink this at least two times every day.
5. You can also eat fresh curry leaves two times a day to reduce the sugar level in your body.
6. Fish-berry is crushed and soaked in water for one day and the juice is taken as the first thing in the morning.

And some more home remedies for diabetes:

- Boil 1 cup of water with 1 teaspoon of cinnamon, cool and drink daily.
- Soak almonds in water and eat every morning before you eat anything else.
- Boil a cup of water with mango leaves; drink the water every morning to treat diabetes.
- A good treatment is to eat soybeans.
- Eat cucumbers daily.
- Exercise to keep your body balanced.
- Add turmeric powder to your food it's good for diabetes and add flavor.
- Eat tomatoes every day.

NATURAL REMEDIES FOR ASTHMA THAT ARE SIMPLE AND EFFECTIVE

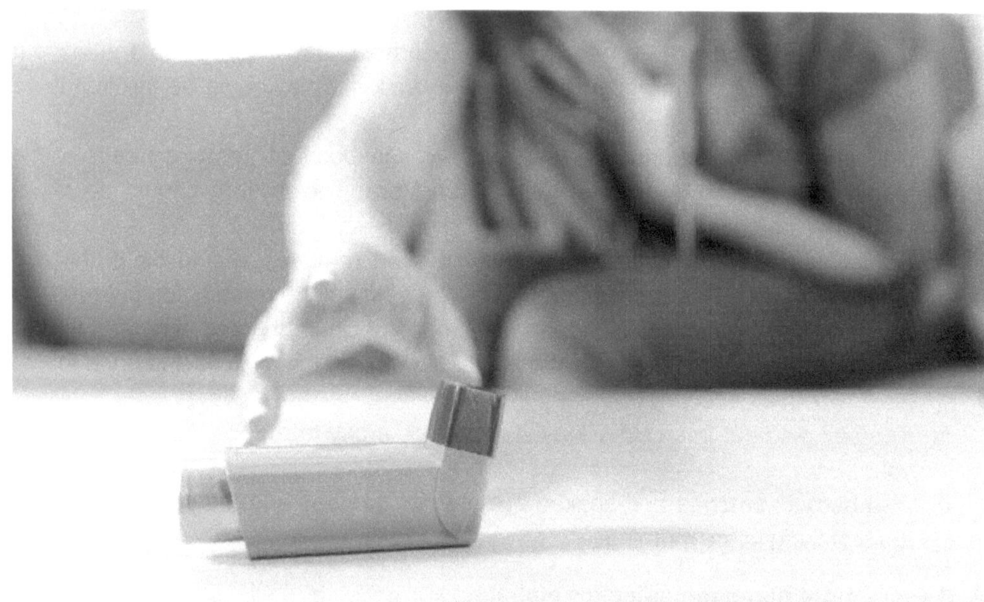

Major causes of asthma

Factors that precipitate an asthma attack are referred to as triggers. They cause the air passages to get clogged and constricted, making it difficult for the patient to breathe. The inflamed bronchioles generate more mucus and also cause the muscles around them to tighten and get irritated, constricting the airways. This is called bronchospasm.

Below are some common causes of asthma -

1. Allergy: For most, it is an allergy to foods, pollens, perfumes, body sprays, deodorizers, the weather, drugs or any other irritants. They vary from person to person. However, dust allergies seem to be the most common factor.
2. Combination of Factors: For others, it is triggered off by a combination of allergic and non-allergic factors including stress and tension, air pollution or infections.
3. Heredity: In most of the cases it has been found that when one or both parents suffer from asthma, the children have similar allergic reactions.
4. Abnormal Body Chemistry: Asthma may result from the abnormal body chemistry involving the body's enzymes or a defect in muscular action within the lungs.

Natural remedies for asthma

Most medication for treating asthma seeks to reduce the inflammation by using anti-inflammatory medications, or inhalers to temporarily dilate the passageway. There are some natural remedies for asthma that helps to lower the frequency of asthmatic episodes. While asthma cannot be cured, it can be managed through appropriate asthma treatment. The first step in asthma treatment involves changing an asthmatic's environment. This type of asthma treatment can be as simple and effective too. This includes washing bedding every week in hot water or eliminating pets from the home.

Another effective asthma treatment involves replacing carpeting with hardwood or tile, using leather or vinyl furniture rather than upholstered chairs and sofas, using the air conditioner and replacing down bedding with bedding made with synthetic materials.

Note: Remember these natural remedies can't replace your asthma medication but can only support your treatment.

NATURAL REMEDY FOR ECZEMA - HOME MADE CLEANSER STOPS THE ITCH AND REDNESS WITHOUT ANY CHEMICALS

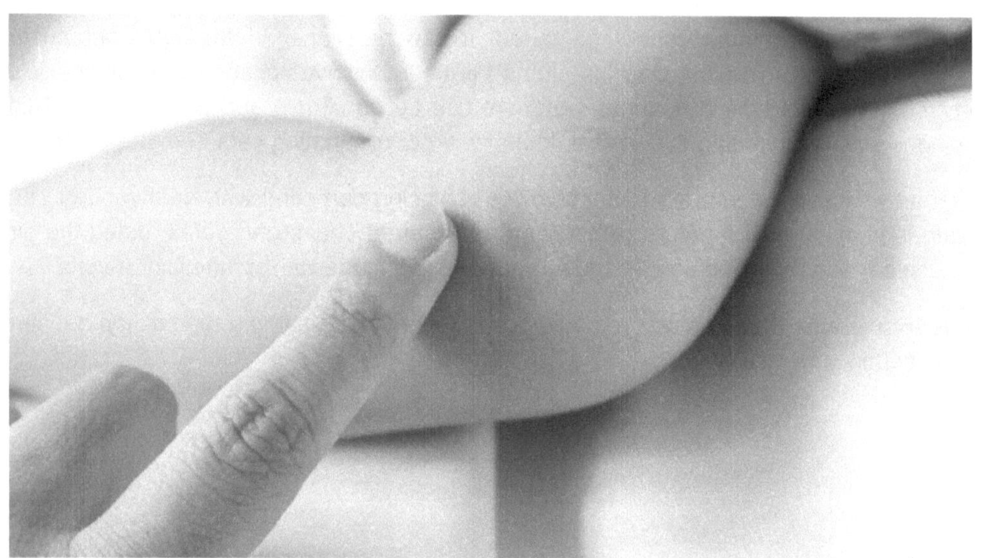

Anyone who has ever suffered from eczema knows how terrible this skin disorder can be. The itch and the scaling are terrible and irritating, not to mention embarrassing and uncomfortable. Just trying to go around doing your usual chores can be a problem because of the pain. The chemical treatments are expensive and take a lot of time to show little results, and usually, eczema just comes back.

One important step in your healing process is proper cleansing. By now, you know better than to try to use commercial formulas, full of chemicals and perfumes that only irritate your skin, and make the problem worse. Here you will find a cleanser made of only natural ingredients that are easy to do and gentle on your skin.

The ingredients you will need are comfrey root, slippery elm bark, and white oak bark to create this natural remedy. Let me explain to you what each of these does and why you have to include them.

1. Comfrey root

Comfrey root helps with reducing the inflammation which in turn reduces the redness of the skin. This will help you stimulate the growth of new cells.

2. White oak bark

This is a natural source of zinc, that helps soothes the skin, and also contains vitamin B12, it also helps reduce the inflammation.

3. Slippery elm bark

Slippery elm bark contains Tannins, which act as natural antibiotics due to its astringent qualities. It will help you prevent infections and reduce the swelling.

Preparation of the Cleanser

- You will need 1 spoon of comfrey root, slippery elm bark and white oak bark for every 2 cups of water. You can use more if you wish to have a larger preparation ready to use.
- Let The ingredients boil and then simmer for 30 minutes. Let the mix cool down and remove any solids.
- Once it is cool, you can use it as you would any other skin cleanser.

KEY NATURAL REMEDIES FOR GOUT THAT ARE ESSENTIAL TO KNOW

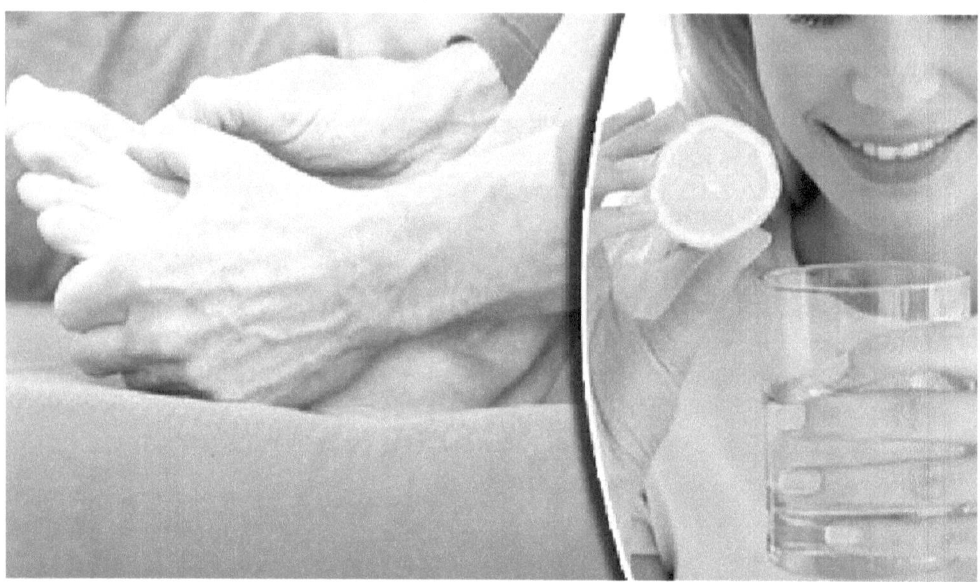

One of the main problems with pharmaceutical drugs rather than using natural remedies for gout is that most of these drugs do not cure gout, but instead simply mask the pain and discomfort. In some cases the lack of pain fools people into thinking that they can use the affected joint instead of resting it, thereby causing even more damage and pain later on.

As you may already know if you have an understanding of what causes gout is that the problem is developed by the build-up of tiny uric acid crystals in body joints caused by high levels of uric acid in the body. Natural remedies for gout addresses this problem by decreasing the uric acid levels in the blood which in turn will diminish the build-up of the pain-causing uric acid crystals.

Another advantage of going with natural remedies for gout is that your gout treatment plan focuses on common sense foods and lifestyle changes such as following a gout diet and knowing the foods to avoid with gout rather than relying on pain-killers and other artificial means as a treatment of gout.

Many of the natural remedies for gout form the basis for most of the gout home remedies that have become very popular online and in bookstores in recent years.

Key Natural Remedies for Gout Prevention

1. Drink lots of water

As already mentioned, high levels of uric acid in the bloodstream lead to gout, so it stands to reason that one of the best natural remedies for gout would be water. Drinking lots of water helps to flush the uric acid from the body avoiding the crystal build-up in joints.

2. Vitamin C

Vitamin C helps to lower the level of uric acid in the body and should be taken daily. Current research indicates 500-3000 mg of Vitamin C should be taken on a daily basis, with additional dosages taken during severe gout attacks.

3. Diet Changes

Eliminating or decreasing the intake of red meat, especially organ meats (heart, liver) that contain high levels of purines is often mentioned as an important part of any natural remedies for gout strategy. When the body breaks down the purines, one of the by-products is uric acid. To reduce the red meat intake and you reduce the production of uric acid.

4. Berry Power

Berries, especially strawberries, are very effective natural remedies for gout because they can actually help to neutralize the uric acid in the body.

5. Vitamin B complex

Vitamin B complex aids the body in changing uric acid into a variety of harmless by-products provided you take at least 350 mg of the Vitamin B complex daily.

6. Apple Cider Vinegar and Honey

The mixture of apple cider vinegar mixed with honey and consumed daily is one of the very popular remedies for gout both for prevention and on-going natural gout treatment.

Popular Natural Remedies for Gout Treatment

This article would not be complete without mentioning a few remedies for gout treatment to help relieve pain and discomfort.

1. Ice

Perhaps the easiest of the natural remedies for gout pain is the application of ice to the swollen and painful areas. Crush the ice and place it into a waterproof bag. Lay a towel over the joint prior to applying the ice pack.

2. Cold Cabbage Leaves

Any discussion of natural remedies for gout treatment wouldn't be complete without mentioning the use of cold cabbage leaves to help reduce gout pain. Simply apply the frozen cabbage leaves to the affected area.

3. Spearmint

Create a poultice made of spearmint and smear it directly onto the swollen joint region is a popular gout treatment if you are into natural remedies for gout as opposed to using commercial products.

There are certainly many more natural remedies for the prevention and treatment for gout than what has been discussed here. The important "take away" from this discussion is the fact that you do not need to feel dependent on prescription drugs to alleviate your symptoms of gout when there is such a wide range of natural remedies for gout available.

DANDRUFF DISASTER - AT HOME ALL NATURAL REMEDIES

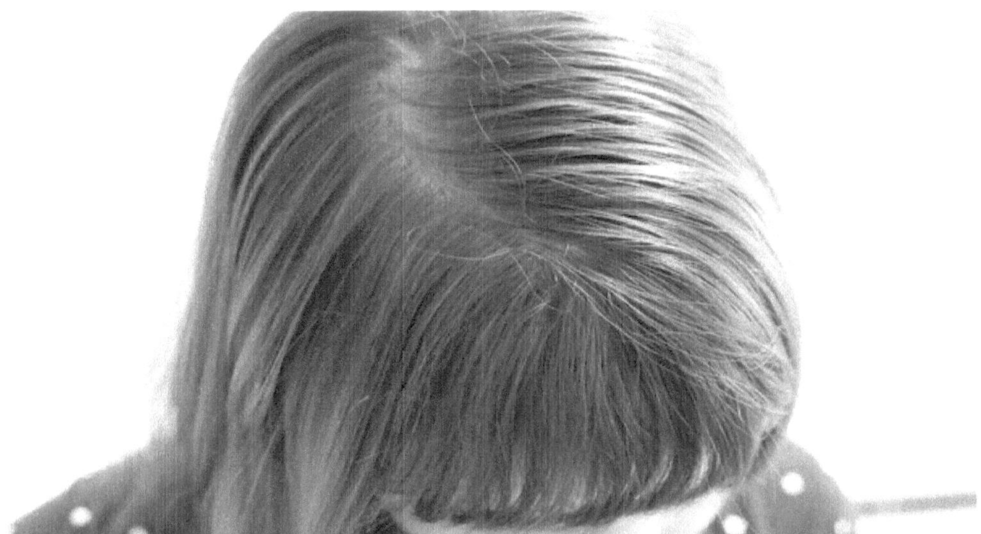

With the problem of dandruff becoming more common as well as more embarrassing, people have begun to think outside the box when it comes to possible cures. When we looked around a little bit, we found a few remedies that not only stood out but seemed to be used by multiple people so we thought they may be worth sharing. First of all, it seems that everyone suffering from bad dandruff has the same embarrassed perspective; most people find it humiliating and are willing to go to the greatest lengths to get rid of it.

Perhaps the most peculiar of the all-natural dandruff cures we found, was the honey yogurt challenge. This one not only seemed strange but somehow people tended to find it effective. By mixing a couple drops of lemon juice with a bit of honey, and adding yogurt, people found a decrease in the amount of dandruff they saw. Just make sure when attempting this all-natural dandruff cure that you don't use too much honey, you don't want a bigger mess than you started with.

Another good idea, that seemed more rational and like something that was done often, was a hot oil massage treatment for the scalp. A lot of people raved of how it not only got rid of their dandruff but made their hair soft and shiny as well. Some even said this left their hair "feeling" healthier.

Don't think that's all though, we heard one more all-natural dandruff curing idea worth sharing with you. This one starts with an egg, one egg, and baby oil. After washing you're advised to scramble the two and leave it on your head to set, in the morning you should wash it with shampoo. While this all-natural dandruff cure may sound gross, it just might work. However, you can take it off within an hour.

BEST NATURAL REMEDIES FOR WRINKLES

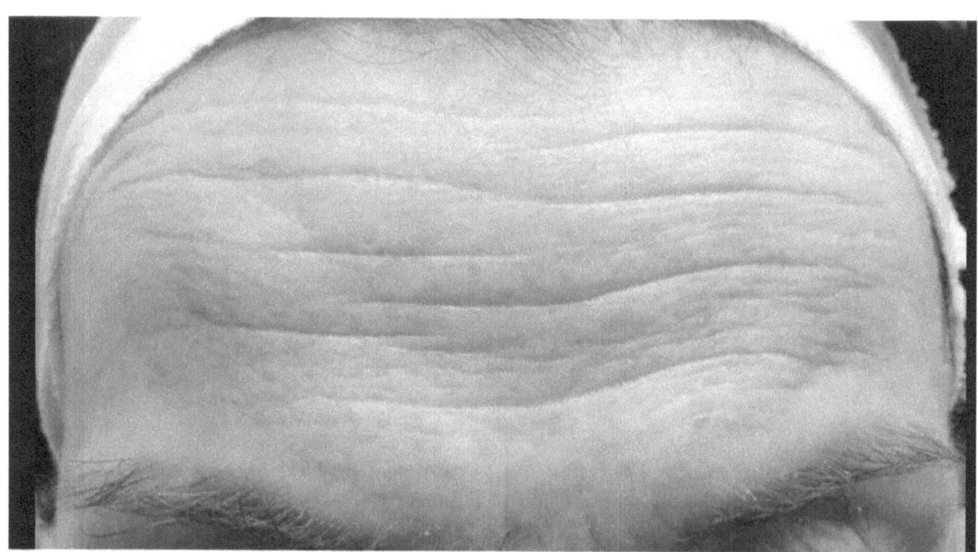

If you are approaching your 30s or 40s you may be already concern about unwanted facial lines and wrinkles, you don't live to look older than your age and you want to look younger, many products and anti-aging treatments exist but most of them are risky, expensive and are not natural or good for your skin health.

The best way to remove wrinkles is to use natural remedies that will create long-lasting results and not just a quick fix. There are natural home remedies that people have used for centuries, natural treatments, natural creams and important healthy lifestyle rules that you should follow.

- ❖ Home remedies for wrinkles can be for example applying cucumbers on your eyes for 15 minutes to reduce wrinkles around the eyes.
- ❖ Vitamins are great for your skin, take B complex vitamins included in beef, eggs, chicken and whole wheat. Antioxidants are also very important, vitamins A, C, and E gives the skin a healthy look and protect it from free radicals.
- ❖ Another home remedy is to make a mixture of honey, olive oil, cream and apply it on the face.
- ❖ To take off blemishes and wrinkles apply lemon juice many times a day.
- ❖ Message the skin with pure castor oil it helps to prevent wrinkles.
- ❖ Those are some natural remedies for wrinkles that are used by many people, you should also take preventive measures to avoid the formation of wrinkles.

- ❖ Avoid smoking and drinking too much alcohol
- ❖ Use sunscreen to protect your skin from the UV rays of the sun.
- ❖ Drink a lot of water every day.
- ❖ And use a good anti-wrinkle cream only if is made of natural ingredients.
- ❖ A good anti-wrinkle cream can be very good to reduce wrinkles gradually if it's made of organic ingredients. For example CynergyTk will increase collagen on the body thus firming the skin and recovering its elasticity. Other ingredients like Coenzyme Q10 are very effective as antioxidants that prevent free radical damage.

HOW TO ALLEVIATE VAGINAL ODOR ON YOUR OWN - NATURAL REMEDIES GUARANTEED TO GET RID OF FEMININE SMELL

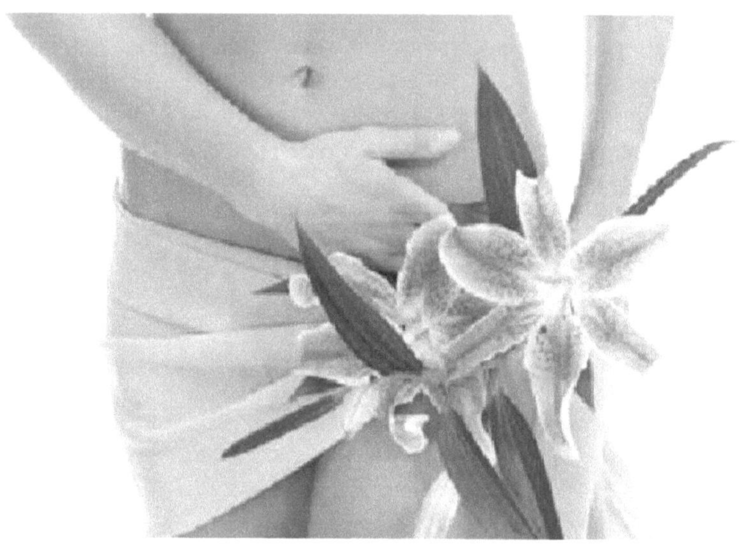

Vaginal odor is easily one of the most embarrassing problems that a woman is forced to deal with in her life. Nothing is quite as embarrassing as the vagina producing a fishy odor. This makes any woman feel dirty and ashamed of her body. You don't want to feel this way anymore. You want to be able to love your body and to be proud of it. It's time that you made this happen for yourself.

In order to alleviate vaginal odor, you don't necessarily have to run to a doctor for relief. You can get relief right from the comfort of your own home. You just need to learn more about some natural remedies guaranteed to get rid of the feminine smell.

Natural remedies work really well for two reasons; they are safe and they are very effective. The more natural a treatment is, the easier your body responds to it. As well, when you use a natural remedy, you allow your body to fight off the infection too. This makes your immune system much stronger and in fact, it actually helps you in the long run. Now you have built up a natural immunity to the problem and you will be able to fight off vaginal odor faster and prevent it better.

One of the best ways to alleviate vaginal odor on your own is to use baking soda. Right now, your vagina is extremely acidic and that is one of the main reasons for the fishy odor. You need to counteract this smell and the best way to do that is to neutralize it with something alkaline. The best way to go about doing this is to use baking soda. All you need is a small amount and some water. You can use this to insert it directly into your body or you can drink it. Either way, baking soda will work to neutralize some of the smell and help to give you relief.

Another way to get rid of feminine smell at home with natural remedies is to up your intake of vitamin C. You have an infection in your body and your white blood cells need to attack it. The only way that you can really make this happen is to boost your white blood cell count by boosting your immune system. Vitamin C can do just that. It is really easy to increase your vitamin C intake because there are so many sources of making that happen. You can drink orange juice or eat more fruits and vegetables. No matter what method you choose, just make sure you are increasing your vitamin C so you can fight off the smell faster.

There is no need for medications or messy creams when you can get relief from vaginal odor fast, right from the comfort of your home.

QUICK HOME-MADE ACNE REMEDIES - EFFECTIVE ACNE SCAR REMOVAL

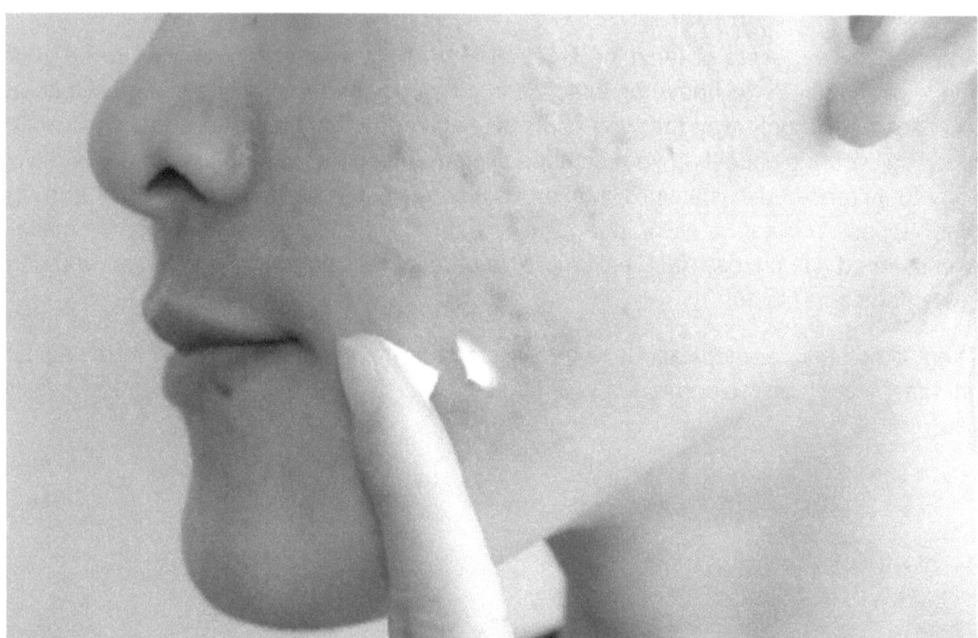

If you are looking for some less expensive and effective ways to get rid of acne scars, then the best way is to use some quick home-made acne remedies.

Many people are tired of trying different methods of removing horrible scars that are caused by this dreadful skin condition. If you are facing a similar situation, then there is no need to despair as there are plenty of options that are available to help you get out of this situation. You can try using some quick remedies which are effective and easy on your pocket as well.

You can find most of the ingredients used for these remedies very easily in your kitchen. The best part about using these remedies is that they are free from harmful chemicals and 100% natural so you need not be worried about any kind of side effects.

However, there is a better solution than using these quick homemade acne remedies - and this involves using effective products like Acnezine, which offers you a complete solution to get rid of all your acne-related problems. Acnezine is made using high-quality natural ingredients, which helps in treating acne outbreaks and blemishes without causing any harm to your skin.

Some quick remedies

❖ One of the quickest remedies that you can make at home is mixing equal quantities of lemon juice and rose water to prepare a solution. Apply this solution on the acne-affected areas, leave it for about 30 minutes, and then clean it using warm water. This is a simple but effective remedy that really works to remove clogged up pores.

❖ Another effective acne scar removal method is to simply use raw potato slices by cutting them into thin slices and rubbing the flat edge over your acne-affected skin. This acts as a wonderful remedy for controlling acne by helping in removing the dead skin and breaks down the bacteria present in the pores.

❖ Cucumber masks can be used as an effective remedy for treating acne and eliminating clogged pores. For this purpose, you need a few pieces of chopped cucumber, which can be made into a puree using a blender. Just keep the puree in the fridge so that it is chilled and you can apply it to your face.

If these acne remedies do not remove your acne scars, then try using Acnezine, which has apparently helped many people to get rid of scar marks and blemishes in a fast and cost-effective manner.

DISCOVERING THE BEST HOME MADE REMEDIES FOR HEARTBURN

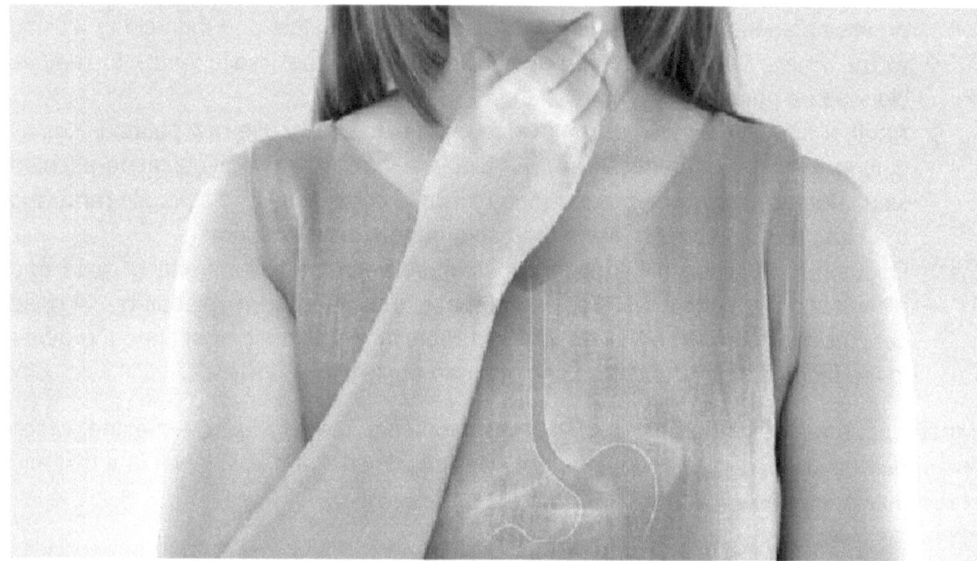

Discovering the best homemade remedies for heartburn is made easy just right here. People are always looking for homemade remedies for heartburn. It is a very common condition that anyone can experience at any stage of their life.

Our stomach needs acids to digest the foods that we eat, but sometimes the acids in the stomach get refluxed upwards to the esophagus which gives a very discomforting sensation of burning in the chest, throat and a sore taste in the mouth. The symptoms may differ depending upon how severe your heartburn condition is.

There are several homemade remedies for heartburn, some of them are;

- ❖ **Vinegar:** one of the most popular homemade remedies for heartburn is vinegar. Use a couple of teaspoons of vinegar in your food. For example, if you are eating chicken, add vinegar to it. Vinegar acts fast as it is acidic in nature and adds to the bulk of acid in the digestive system and helps indigestion.
- ❖ **Apple:** apples are very good if eaten in heartburn condition. Apples also help to control the acidic functions taking place in the digestive system.
- ❖ **Chewing gums:** homemade remedies for heartburn also include chewing gum. Some people might not agree, but it really cure heartburn, it helps in reducing the burning sensation in the chest and throat to a great extent.
- ❖ **Baking soda:** baking soda is regarded as a heartburn remedy because it contains sodium bicarbonate, which is an alkali, the opposite of acid, which is the main cause of heartburn. Pour one teaspoon of baking soda into a full glass of

water and drink it. The solution neutralizes the acidity in the stomach hence, heartburn sensation is stopped immediately. Caution; do not take if you have high blood pressure.

❖ **Green leafy Vegetables:** green leafy vegetables contain a high amount of fibers, which eases the digestion process. Include green leafy vegetables in your salads and food on a regular basis in every meal, especially if you suffer from chronic acid reflux and heartburn.

Other than these homemade remedies for heartburn, you should also avoid certain foods and ingredients that may aggravate the heartburn condition. There are certain foods that trigger the illness which should be avoided or eliminated completely from your diet plan. Restrict or avoid beverages containing caffeine like tea, coffee, soft drinks. Consumption of alcohol should also be restricted or completely avoided. Stay away from mint foods as the mint itself causes heartburn. Furthermore, avoid citrus fruits like lemon, oranges, which may build up acid content in your stomach. Tomato and tomato-based products also may influence acid reflux in the stomach.

So, if you avoid foods that are considered to induce heartburn and follow natural homemade remedies for heartburn you can minimize your heartburn symptoms.

NATURAL WAYS TO EASE THE DISCOMFORT FROM A COLD

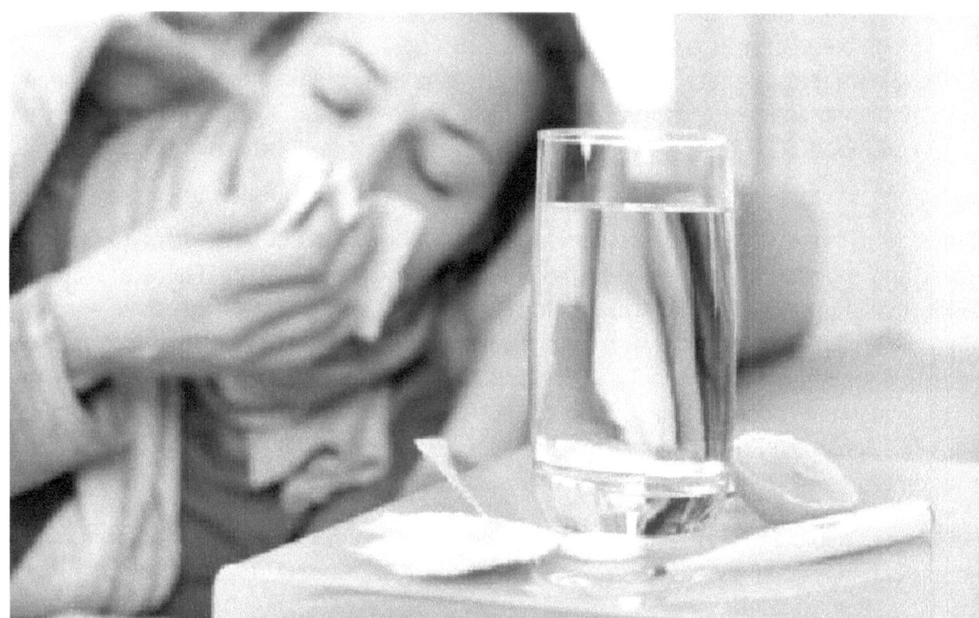

While we call it the common cold, the actual illness is usually some variation of a rhinovirus. That's why it's so easy to catch the next one. Like the flu, they can mutate and any immunity factors would be gone.

Dealing with the cold is another matter entirely. Most of them produce the same symptoms, runny nose, congestion, coughing, etc. Fortunately, if you have a relatively well-stocked pantry and fridge, you can make your own remedies.

1. **Congestion:** Pressure in the sinuses and the inability to breathe through the nose is one of the most frustrating aspects of having a cold. For this, I like to start with steam. You can sit in the bathroom with the shower on hot, use a hot vaporizer or an old trick my mother taught me. Bring one part vinegar to three parts water to a boil. Once it starts steaming, hold your head over it and breathe it in. This requires some care, as if you knock the pan off the stove you could get burnt.

2. **Coughing:** The coughing associated with the cold is usually part of a postnasal drip. Simple cough syrup may be all that's needed. Mix equal parts honey and lemon juice. Adults can handle a tablespoon, but a teaspoon may be better for children. Never give honey to children under two.

3. **Headache:** If it feels like the pressure over your eyes is threatening to push those needful things out, you have what is called a sinus headache. To be

honest, an over the counter pain reliever is your best bet, but while you're waiting for it to work, get a cloth and dampen it with cool water. Lie down in a darkened room and lay it on your forehead. Turn it over each time it seems to get warm. That will help reduce the swelling and pressure.

4. **Runny Nose:** While this is preferable to having a stopped up nose, one can quickly feel like Rudolph the Red-Nosed Reindeer if something isn't done. Many people cannot take decongestants, particularly if they have high blood pressure. However, lemon balm and sage could offer some relief, as can the steam treatments.

5. **Sore Throat:** This can be helped by the honey/lemon mixture suggested for coughs, but if it is really sore, you may need something else. A combination of cinnamon, whole cloves, and whole allspice may do the trick. Simmer them on the stove for about twenty minutes and drink about half a cup. If you are diabetic, you may want to skip the cinnamon as it could affect sugar levels.

CHILDREN'S COLDS - KIDS AND COMMON COLDS EXPLAINED

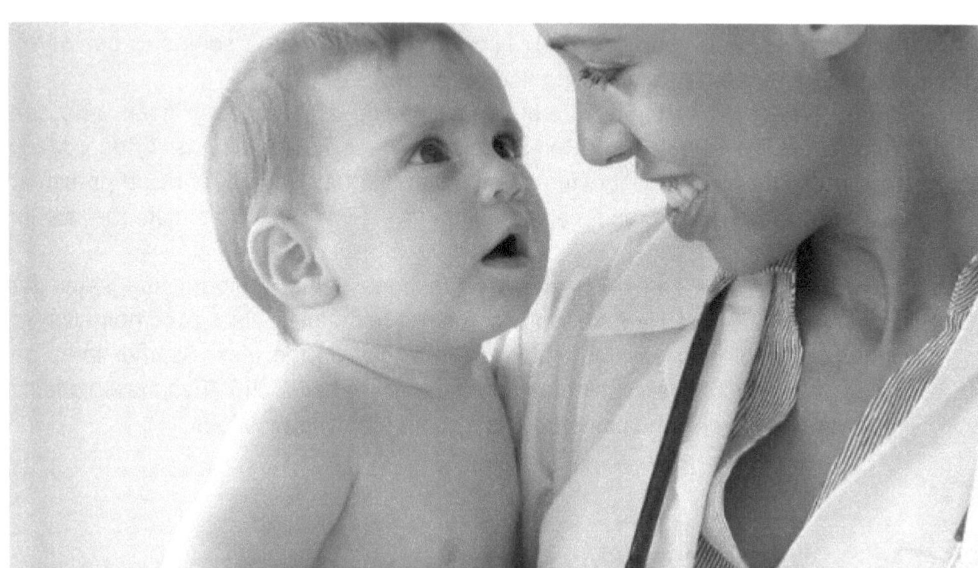

It can be scary when your child catches a cold, or anything debilitating, but if you know what you're dealing with, then you'll know how to make the right choices and do everything you can to help your child get well soon. Here's everything you need to know about cases of flu, colds, and kids.

The Common Cold

The average child catches about six to twelve colds a year. Some minor, some more serious. So when your kid gets sick, it doesn't mean you're a bad parent, it means that your kid is, well, just a kid. Kids get sick a lot because their bodies are still developing-their immune systems are still learning how to deal with these viruses and as we all know, kids typically don't wash their hands as regularly as most adults.

In other words, they call it the "common cold" because it's really quite common.

The cold is a viral infection affecting the upper respiratory tract and can be contracted from just about anywhere. Interestingly, it was Benjamin Franklin who first noted the contagious nature of the cold, which is impressive when you consider that viruses hadn't even been discovered at that point. Franklin pointed out that the cold seemed to pass from person to person when they shared small rooms together or talked closely while at a party. About one hundred and fifty years later, science proved Franklin right.

Symptoms of a cold include sore throat, runny nose, fever, headache, coughing, sneezing, and stuffy nose.

As they say "there's no cure for the common cold," but there are treatment and prevention. It's interesting to note that alcohol and anti-bacterial soap actually don't do much to kill the virus off. Using plain old soap and water, on the other hand, is an effective way to physically remove the virus from the surface of the skin.

You can use analgesics, cough medicine, chest rub vapors, and saltwater gargling to treat the symptoms of the cold, but there's no known treatment to shorten the span of the illness. Luckily, the disease is self-limiting and will typically clear itself up in about a week.

The Flu

Almost everyone has suffered the flu a few times in their lives, but it can be at its scariest when it happens to kids. Children seem to suffer a lot more than adults under the physically taxing symptoms of the flu.

These symptoms include fatigue, fever, chills, coughing, general pain, weakness and discomfort, and various cold-like symptoms including runny nose, headaches, sore throat, and so on. While the flu is often mistaken for a cold (and vice versa), the flu is actually much more serious than even the roughest colds. Flu sickness involves muscle pains and digestion problems that the cold can't come close to replicating.

Interestingly, the flu virus, influenza, is not responsible for the so-called "24-hour flu" which is not flu at all, but gastroenteritis.

Influenza is spread essentially the same way as the cold, though-it easily contracted when sharing living ⬚uarters with one who has the flu, talking closely, or rubbing your hands around your mouth or eyes without having recently washed.

Influenza is also contracted through direct contact with unsanitary surfaces. For instance, direct contact with bird droppings can lead to the flu. Still, most cases of the flu begin with "aerosol", or airborne viruses.

Luckily, the flu is almost never terminal, in spite of what the media might have you believe. Most cases of flu, even the most serious, won't kill anyone who is of relatively good health.

Flu season lasts through the winter, which seems odd, considering that colds can occur all year round. The more common prevalence of the flu in colder weather seems to be caused by the drier air and the fact that people spend more time indoors when the weather outside is disagreeable. Spending a lot of time cooped up is bad for your immune system and overall health.

HOW TO BOOST THE IMMUNE SYSTEM OF YOUR BABY AND TODDLER NATURALLY

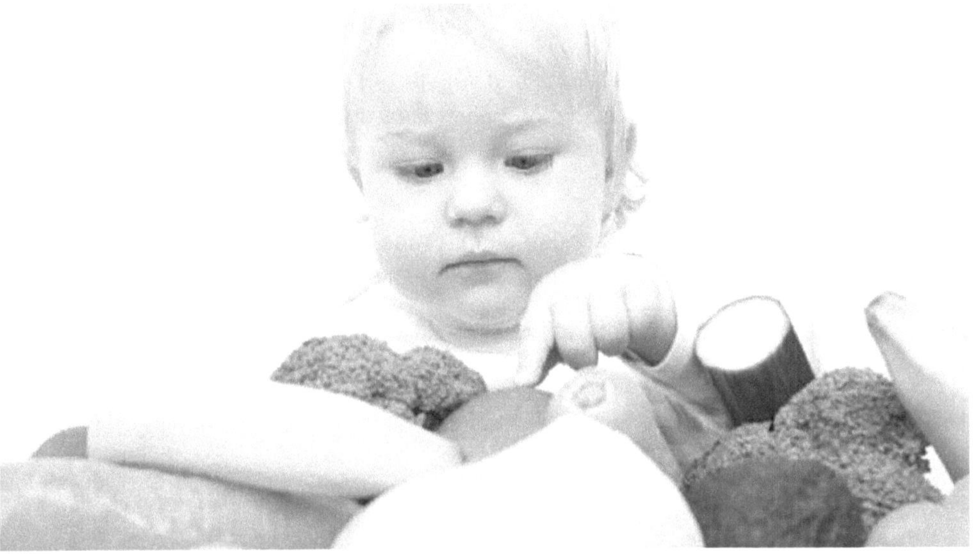

Young infants are less able to fight any infection as their immune systems are still immature. We always try to protect our babies and toddlers from infection and build their immunity through vaccination. But vaccination alone cannot fight off all kinds of diseases like common cold, flu, etc. It is a fact that healthy diet, exercise, and cleanliness can ward off various disease-causing bacteria, viruses, and other germs.

Natural and herbal remedies, prepared at home, can also relieve them from the discomfort and suffering of the disease.

Ways to boost the immune system of the babies and toddlers

- ❖ Healthy Diet
- ❖ Exercise
- ❖ Hygiene
- ❖ Natural Remedies

A healthy diet boosts immune response

Breast milk is not only rich in all kinds of nutrients but also provides immune protection against diseases. It is the richest and only source of antibodies for the babies who solely thrive on breastfeeding. No commercial formula can provide the antibodies that are present in breast milk that wards off various infections.

A diet rich in complex carbohydrates like whole grains, and plenty of fruits and vegetables, proteins, is best to support a healthy immune system. Cut down on refined foods like sugar is also suggested. Whole foods like brown rice, whole wheat products provide steady increase in energy and stimulate the immune response of the body.

Give your babies different colored fruits and vegetables to eat which are rich in immune-boosting carotenoids and flavenoids. Veggies like carrot, green beans, raw papaya, white potato, sweet potato, pumpkins, etc. are good for babies who have started to eat solids.

Fruits like banana, apple, pear, apricot, plum, prune, and melon are also good. Fruits rich in vitamin C, like the citrus fruits and berries, etc. aid in the immune response.

Garlic, onion, and thyme have antiviral qualities. These can be added in a little amount to the baby's food after 10 to 12 months of age.

An increase in fluid intake during cold, fever, flu or diarrhea provides healing support.

Offer a lot of proteins in the form of full cream milk, chicken and fish to provide all the essential amino acids required by the body.

Exercise will keep them fit

We all know that a good diet is a big boost to the immunity of your child but we do not often think of exercise as a help in this endeavor. It is a fact that exercise not only helps to get more oxygen and helps to remove harmful toxins from the body but also stimulates to release certain chemicals in the body, which helps the immune system fight bacteria.

Young infants cannot exercise as old kids but we can always engage them in various kinds of physical activities that would give the same result. Let the toddlers go outside and help them run around. Do not let them sit in front of the TV. A few hours of active play will keep them fit and healthy.

Maintaining hygiene keeps the family happy

Always wash your hands before handling the baby because good handwashing can remove the germs from our hands. The golden rule is to wash your hands with any kind of soap for about 15 seconds.

Avoid people who are most likely to be sick like those with fevers, runny nose or coughs, and also other children who are the most common carrier of different contagious forms of germs. Maintaining cleanliness and hygiene at home can keep the baby and the family healthy and happy.

Natural Remedies

There are several natural things that you can buy or prepare at home to improve the immune response of the body and make the baby or the toddler feel better when they are sick.

Eucalyptus oil: If your baby is suffering from cold, fever and body ache put a few drops of Eucalyptus oil in a handkerchief and let the young one smell it. Keep it beside the pillow when he or she sleeps. Eucalyptus fights infection, kills bacteria, and opens the sinuses to drain. This works amazingly well.

Cinnamon Oil: You can massage a drop of Cinnamon oil mixed with olive oil on the bottom of the feet, which is good for boosting the immune system and fighting viruses. Do not put it on the skin of the face, arms or legs; otherwise, it can burn the skin. The skin under the feet is tougher.

Fennel Tea: Prepare fennel tea with one teaspoon of fennel per cup of boiling water, boil for 20 minutes and give two spoons of the tea three times a day to help break up mucus.

Fennel Water: Fennel water is similar to anise and dill water. This is used to ease flatulence in infants. Syrup made from fennel can be used to treat babies with colic or painful teething.

There is nothing harder to watch your baby suffer from a disease. Some simple precautions and practices can boost their immune system and keep them healthy happy and smiling.

HOW TO EASE THE SYMPTOMS OF THE FLU IN CHILDREN

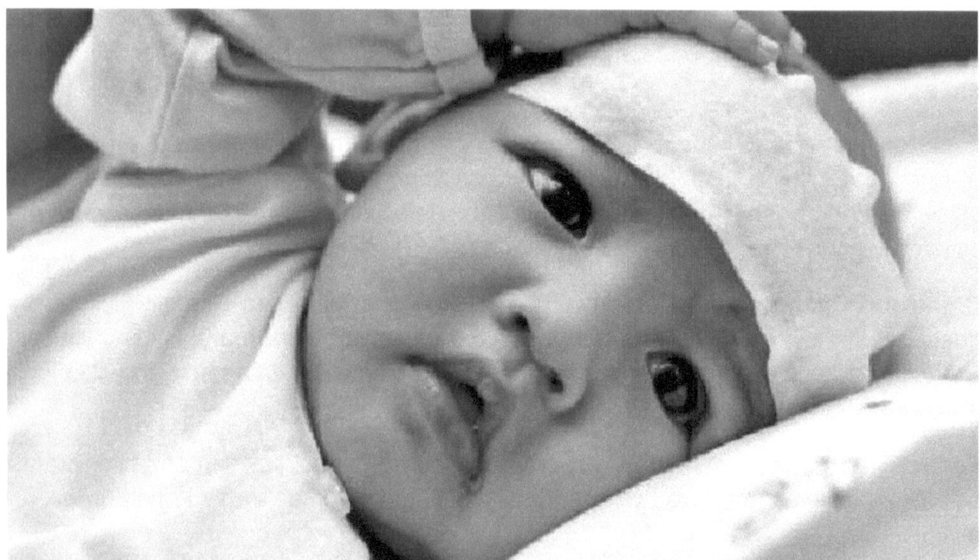

When it comes to the flu, there is a world of difference between children and adults. Many things we might be able to take are dangerous to children. There are also things that are safe for older children that can't be used on or around younger ones. It can be like a minefield. Add to that the natural stress you feel as a parent, it has the makings of a nightmare.

There are things you can do, though they should be coordinated through your pediatrician's office. These suggestions may be very beneficial used under the right circumstances.

Herbally speaking, a lot of caution should be used for anyone under eighteen. The younger the child, the more caution you should exercise. Age limits currently available will be included in this list.

Catnip: The flu makes all of us restless, but children seem to have the worst of it. They don't understand the feeling and they don't know how to address it. Catnip is a mild nervine that can help your child rest better. Don't give it to children under two. Consult the pediatrician for children under six, but older children should tolerate it fairly well.

Cinnamon Tea: This preparation can help you sweat, a traditional treatment for any virus. It is believed that you can "sweat out" the illness. This is very strong and should not be given to children under fourteen without the consent of the pediatrician. If your child is a diabetic, don't use it as it could cause a sharp drop in blood sugar.

Chamomile: The slightly apple-scented flowers of this plant make a relaxant, to help induce sleep. It should be safe for children ten and older. Check with the doctor for those under that age.

Eucalyptus: The information about this common cold/flu remedy may surprise you. Children two and under should have no contact with this herb, either in a vapor, essential oil or in cough remedies. Children under six can handle the rub and oil, but should not be given any oral remedies...including cough drops...that contain this potent herb. For those older children, it may be very useful. It can help soothe a cough, open up nasal passages and help clear the chest.

Honey/Lemon: One of the easiest cough and sore throat remedies you may be able to give your kids. Mix a fifty/fifty combination together and give one tablespoon at a time. Children two and under should not be given honey.

Peppermint: My second favorite herb is peppermint. It can do a lot of good things, including stop a cough, ease a sore throat and help an upset stomach. However, don't give it to children two or under. Don't use anything with the essential oil in it, either. This can cause a serious breathing disorder in very young children.

Wild Cherry Bark: Did you ever wonder why so many cough remedies are cherry flavored? There actually is a reason behind it. Cherry bark has been used as a cough suppressant since pre-history. It contains a constituent that changes to cyanide once it hits stomach acid. In small amounts, cyanide is useful in that capacity.

Due to the fact that it is a potentially life-threatening toxin, work with your doctor and a qualified herbal practitioner. As you can imagine, the amount between therapeutic and dead isn't large for small kids.

Non-Herb Remedies

Steam is one of the best things you can use to relieve the congestion caused by the flu bug. There are several applications that may be useful depending on circumstances and the age of the child.

Shower: Turning the shower on hot and sitting with your child in the bathroom may be the simplest remedy. You don't want to put the child in the water, just sit there and let it run.

Vaporizer: These units contain very hot water. Follow all of the safety instructions that come with the unit. If yours is inherited, like mine, look up the precautions needed on-line.

Second, read the ingredients of any products that can be added to it carefully. Most vaporizers have a place where you can put some sort of vapor that will melt and then be added to the steam. As mentioned above, peppermint and eucalyptus should not be used on young children.

Vinegar/Water: You may not be able to get young kids to use this remedy. Also, it could be somewhat dangerous as it is not enclosed like the water in a vaporizer. Put one part vinegar in four parts water, bring to a boil and breathe the steam. Due to the boiling water, use extreme caution with children. It is probably best to use this only on older kids who will be more careful.

How important it is for you to work with your child's doctor when dealing with the flu can never be overemphasized enough. The doctor knows your child's medical history and what he or she is taking. This can make a big difference in choosing which way to deal with the crisis. The doctor will also give you signs to look for that indicate your child is in trouble.

NATURAL REMEDIES TO HELP YOUR CHILD FIGHT COLDS AND FLUS

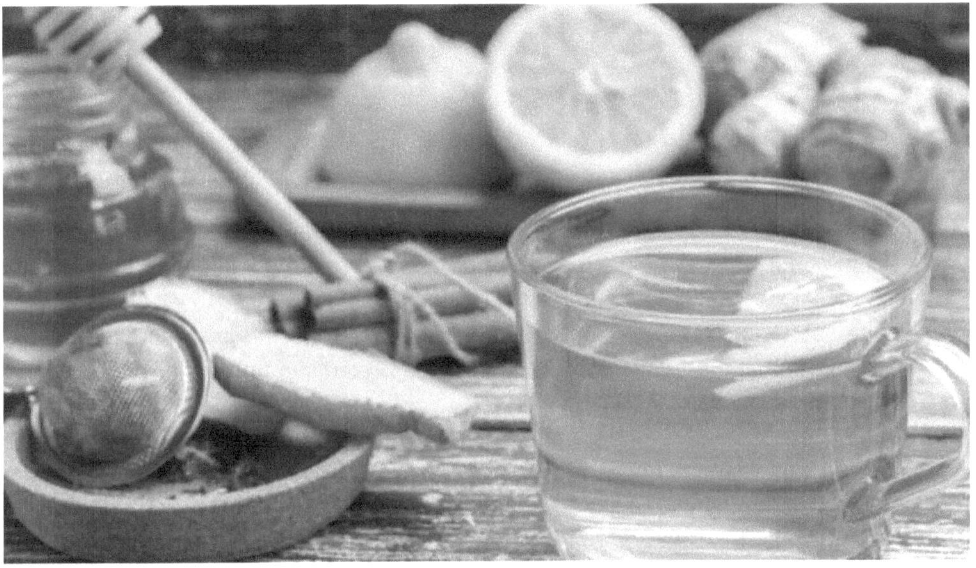

With the school year and fall season in gear, your kids are exposed to more germs and may start coming home with a runny nose and sore throat. What can you do as a parent during this time to help prevent your kids from getting sick, or when they are ill, to alleviate their symptoms and help them get well as quickly as possible?

Prevention

The first line of defense is always prevention. Try these tips to keep your kids healthy when others around them are sick.

- ❖ Make sure your kids are getting plenty of sleep. This is when their body heals and regenerates the most, so getting adequate rest is vital to staying healthy.
- ❖ Try and monitor your kids' stress levels. Stress depresses your immune system, so with increased and sustained levels of stress, there is a greater chance of becoming ill.
- ❖ Have them drink plenty of water. Hydrating keeps toxins from building up in your system and helps to flush them out of the body.
- ❖ Make sure they are playing or exercising regularly. Moving your body increases your circulation, helping to move blood and lymph along. This allows your white blood cells to circulate and fight germs better. Increasing blood flow also flushes toxins away from muscles and organs, and sweating from exercise or play also removes toxins through the skin.

❖ Decrease sugar in the diet. Limit processed foods, pastries, candies, etc. as sugar also impairs the immune system and your overall ability to fight colds and cases of flu.

The Onset Of A Cold Or Flu

Your child comes home feeling a little fatigued and is starting to get congested. What are some things for keeping their illness at bay and speeding up the healing process?

❖ Have your child continue to drink more water and get plenty of rest. These are still the best ways to help support our body's natural defenses and give our body a greater opportunity to fight off any infections.
❖ Take out sugar completely and decrease mucus-producing foods, such as dairy, citrus, and bananas. This will lessen the load on the immune system and prevent any congestion from becoming worse.
❖ Echinacea and elderberry are some great herbs that can help boost the immune system and combat upper respiratory infections. The glycerite forms of these herbs are also tasty for children.
❖ Other herbs that are warming and good for colds and congestion include cinnamon, ginger, cloves, and yarrow. They can increase circulation and help stimulate body heat.
❖ The wet sock treatment is very helpful for increasing circulation and decreasing congestion in the head, throat, and chest. It also helps with sleep and stimulates the immune system.

The Full-Blown Cold Or Flu

Your child now has a full-blown cold or flu. They are tired, congested, have a cough, and are running a fever. What are some extra things or treatments you can add to relieve symptoms?

❖ The same treatments as above can be continued for supporting the immune system.
❖ Chamomile tea is wonderful for children because it relaxes them so they can sleep while also helping to clear coughs and congestion and decreasing fever.
❖ To increase drainage and help relieve congestion, a number of things can help:
❖ Taking horehound and mullein internally is good for clearing bronchial congestion by stimulating coughs. Mullein is also an antimicrobial to help fight infections.
❖ Thyme and Eucalyptus essential oils can be added to 1 ounce of olive oil to rub behind the ears, down the neck, and on the chest, before your child goes to bed or upon waking. The essential oils can also be added to steam showers or a big basin of hot water for your child to inhale to relieve the congestion.

❖ A mustard pack is also great for a congested chest (procedure for a mustard pack found below).

❖ For a dry, spasmodic cough, hyssop and black cherry are great antitussives for children. Soothing throat herbs for dry coughs also include mullein and marshmallow root.

Extended immune support

For kids that may have multiple respiratory infections throughout fall or winter, other supplements to support the immune system can be added.

❖ Vitamin C and zinc stimulate the immune system and help to both prevent and reduce the duration of colds.

❖ Probiotics not only help with gut health, but they also boost our immunity.

❖ Fish oil also helps modulate the immune system and decreases inflammation.

The most important factors for preventing illnesses still center around the basics of rest, hydration, and getting the right nutrients. If your children get these basics, they will be less likely to become sick, but if they do get sick, these natural treatments can help to ease their symptoms as well as expedite their healing process.

Treatments

Wet Sock Treatment

Materials:

+ 1 pair of thin cotton socks in ice water
+ 1 pair of dry, thick wool socks

Right before bed, soak feet in hot water for 5-10 minutes or take a hot shower/bath. Wring out cotton socks and put on feet. Put dry wool socks over the cotton socks, and go to bed with socks on.

Mustard Pack

Materials:

+ 2 pieces of thin cloth (muslin is best or old cut-up T-shirt)
+ 1 tbsp dry mustard powder
+ Flour (adult: 4tbsp, child: 8 tbsp, infant: 12 tbsp)
+ Hot water

Mix flour and mustard. Add enough hot water to make a medium-thin paste. Put one piece of muslin over chest, spread mustard paste thinly over entire cloth, then cover with remaining cloth to make a mustard "sandwich." Put a piece of cling wrap over top and cover with a heating pad or hot water bottle for about 10-20 minutes. The skin should not be red; watch for skin irritation. Clean the area well after treatment.

HOW TO REDUCE PHLEGM AND EXCESS MUCUS

Did you just get over a nasty cold or flu yet still have or feel too much mucus you can't get rid of? Most of us think that mucus is a horrible slime but the truth is we need it in our bodies. In fact, it is a lubricator for our sinus cavities, our guts, and our lungs. It is our protector. Mucus contains antibodies when our bodies are challenged with a virus or bacteria or something we have an allergy too. That gue is a way our body is keeping us healthy. Without it we wouldn't function properly. It is when our bodies go into overdrive that there is a problem.

Most of us know that dairy is a big mucus producer, however did you know that eating eggs, meat, sugar, wheat, processed foods, and certain beverages, grains and nuts can also produce too much mucus?

It is important to evaluate your food intake, its sources, and volume you are taking in to understand this more. When you begin to eliminate or reduce these foods and add in other foods you can experience results.

Too much chicken, eggs, and meats produce too much acid in the body, let alone if they are not organic, these foods will produce even more mucus. Likewise, too many grains can also be problematic. In addition wheat, sugar, certain beverages like coffee can also produce too much mucus. When eating these types of foods choosing organic is best! It is vital to your health!

When choosing proteins aim for plant-based proteins like beans, broccoli, cucumbers, spinach, and much more. It is important to choose healthy plant-based proteins to actually produce good oxygen and circulation in your body and a healthy mucous content.

There are also a variety of lean and grass-fed meats if chosen that are much healthier for you as white fish and healthy forms of soy to give you vitality. After all, you don't want to eat something that has been fed with hormones or something that has been fed GMO diet plans. This can be crucial to your health.

Likewise, too many grains can also be problematic. My advice is to stay with gluten-free grains such as quinoa and millet. Other grains can produce too much mucus as they may have gluten. In addition many of us have too much of a fiesta with grains even healthy ones that if not properly burned will turn into sugar. It is important to eat well balanced and not too much of one thing to avoid allergy and overdrive in your body. It is also very important to exercise!

Sugar holds no nutritional content at all. It tastes good and even smells good! Walking into a candy store or buying fresh baked and yeasty out of the oven loaves of bread, pies, and cookies or dreaming of dancing sugar plums over our heads are fun and addicting, however this can also be a contributing factor why your body is producing too much mucus.

Processed foods and too many wheat products can also cause inflammation. Too much oily nuts such as peanuts and even natural peanut butter can throw off your natural bodies mucus production. It is better to eat roasted nuts in their whole form. If not buying roasted always soak your nuts first before roasting them.

Sugary beverages, too much coffee or even herbal tea containing too much caffeine will also aid in the production of acid throwing off too your natural PH balance. Likewise too much salt can actually upset your natural stomach mucous lining causing things to disarray.

The good thing is by carefully reviewing your diet and what you are eating you will be able to decrease your body's mucous overdrive. By eliminating and reducing some of the foods above, adding in exercise, getting good rest, decreasing stress your body will regain balance again and remember mucus is a good thing just not too much of it!

Get Rid Of Mucus

This mucus is an infection that is caused by bacteria which simply can be due to cold or change in the weather. The mucus is found in sinusitis which is located between your nose and behind your eyes. It is highly irritative as can block your nasal passage and throat cavity. Generally, people face this problem mostly in winter season when you are caught by severe cold and your nose is stuffed with some debris. Sensitive people suffer from some infection with slight change of weather. The debris that creates the blockage is known as mucus. The mucus is common happenings so there is wide assortment of remedy to get rid of mucus. Let's find out how we can tackle mucus in various areas.

How to get rid of mucus in my nose? Well, to overcome the mucus problem in throat I would tell you a home remedy or a natural remedy of mucus. This process is well known as irrigation in which we use the mixture of water and sea salt. The mixture is poured into one nostril and waited till the time this mixture comes out from the other nostril. This seems a quite difficult task, but as you practice you will expertise in it. The treatment is favored for instant relief and that too without any side effect. Furthermore, this curing method is 100% natural and it can be done without getting the help of an expert. Isn't it the easiest way to get rid of mucus?

How to get rid of mucus in the throat? For treatment you just need hot or warm water and inhale its vapors sitting at coach anywhere in your house. It's better if you add little mint or lemon juice in it. Hot vapors have the tendency to thin your mucus. The thinned mucus, later on, will come out from your throat as you cough. This method is also among the best natural cure for sinus infection.

How to get rid of mucus in bronchitis? Our bronchitises are among the significant parts of our body so you can't experiment while treating mucus in bronchitis. The best treatment to cure mucus in bronchitis is by apple cider vinegar juice. Just add 1 or 2 tablespoons of apple vinegar in one cup hot water (bearable) and gulp it and just after the application you will feel it's effect. Mucus from bronchitis will move away.

WHAT FOOD WILL GET RID OF PHLEGM?

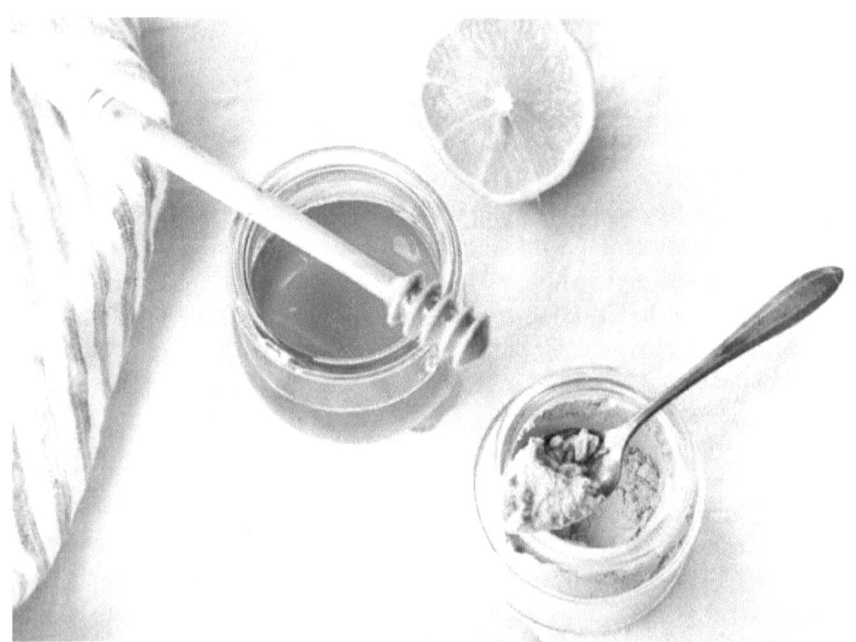

Phlegm is a thick mucus or gel that blocks your throat and nasal passages, usually when there is a viral or bacterial infection in the respiratory system. Your body produces phlegm when there are excessive toxins in your body. The natural reaction is to try to cough it out. However excessive coughing can damage the lining of your throat. Some people prescribe honey & lemon drinks, some take bitter herbs or gargle with salt water when they have a sore throat. What about nuts; some people say they are too dry, but they have many beneficial oils. Which remedy is the best to get rid of phlegm and soothe your throat?

First, honey & lemon both have strong anti-bacterial and anti-viral properties. (Only buy organic honey as most non-organic kinds of honey are processed at high temperatures that kill most of the enzymes in it.) Honey & lemon juice added to boiling water initially soothes the throat then it continues the healing process by killing the virus or bacteria that's causing the mucus.

Traditional Chinese Medicine (TCM) says that excessive phlegm is a condition of the lungs, kidneys, and spleen. When your immune system is weak and cold air enters your lungs or your kidneys the cold moisture in your body condenses and thickens to form phlegm. Bitter herbs and food strengthen your lungs, kidneys, and spleen so that they can work together to get rid of phlegm. Alfalfa, bitter melon, romaine lettuce, citrus rind, asparagus, fennel, and celery are some common vegetables that help loosen phlegm, push it down your throat and through your digestive system to the bowels. Other more potent bitter herbs are chamomile, dandelion (leaf and root), fennel (vegetable and seeds), horseradish, chaparral, burdock, echinacea, and yarrow. Fresh leaves, grated roots or small seeds can be added to salads. Dried leaves, roots and larger seeds can be added to cooking or brewed as a tea. Dandelion root ground up makes a great coffee substitute.

Many nuts are also useful for getting rid of phlegm. Almonds and walnuts are bitter foods that loosen phlegm. They warm the lungs and relieve asthmatic symptoms. Hazelnuts fortify the spleen and give your body more energy to fight disease. Nuts are best roasted on low heat in the oven for about 15 to 20 minutes to bring out their oils and flavor. Once you smell the flavor coming from the oven turn it off. (Any longer you will burn them and dry them out.)

Gargling with salt water or eating sea vegetables loosens phlegm that is sticking to the sides of the throat. The salty flavor partially dissolves the phlegm so that it can be eliminated. Sea vegetables are rich in essential minerals like iodine, calcium, magnesium, and potassium. The mineral salts in sea vegetables work together to mop up toxins in the body (including phlegm) and take them to the bowels.

Other cleansing foods like onions, garlic, kale, cabbage, apples, avocados, grapefruit, and various berries are also great for restoring the nutrient balance of your body then your immune system can function efficiently to get rid of unwanted bacteria. The worst thing you can consume is milk or natural yogurt as these tend to cause more phlegm.

WHAT ARE ESSENTIAL OILS? AN OVERVIEW OF ESSENTIAL OILS

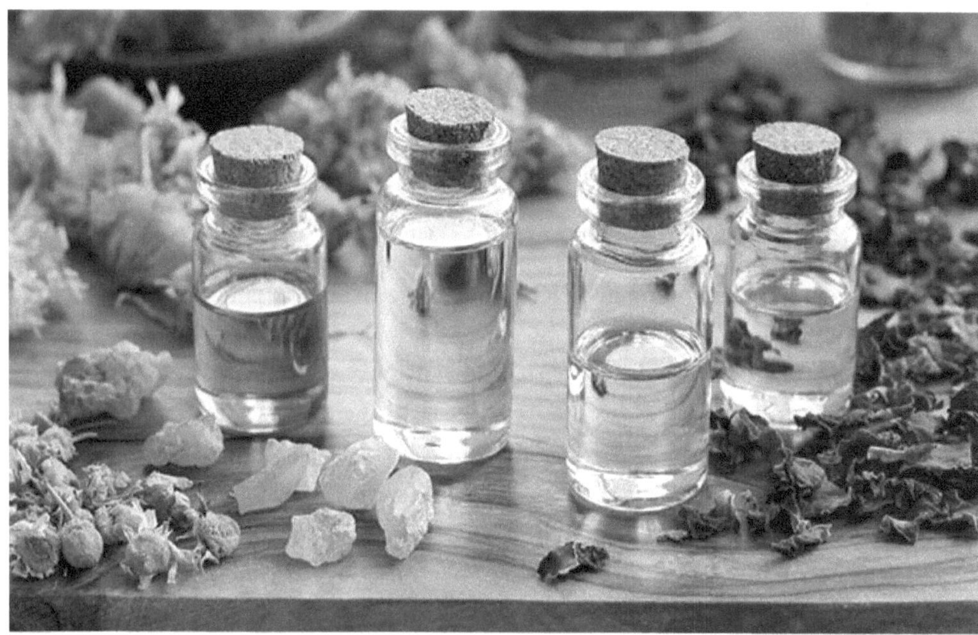

Essential oils are highly concentrated liquids that contain volatile aroma compounds from specific plants. Contrary to being called "oils", they are not oily feeling at all. The majority of them are clear, but there are some that are amber or yellow in color. The color would vary on what type of plant the oil was made from.

These oils are made by extracting them from a particular plant species. They can be extracted from many different parts of the plant, such as the flower, seeds, stems, bark, leaves, roots, and wood of the plant. There are several different methods of extraction, the most common being steam distillation. Some other methods are carbon dioxide extraction, pressing, and solvent extraction.

Essential oils are sold either as pure oil, oil made from only one kind of plant, or as a blend of several different oils. Buying the blended oils saves you from having to buy each one separately and then mixing them yourself. Buying all of the oils individually can be quite pricey, so buying blends can save you money as well as time.

However, the disadvantage is that you have no control over the blend ratios and which oils are used in the blend. Also, by not blending them yourself, the blend can't be reliably mixed with other oils if you don't know what oils were used. Some oils can't be mixed with each other, so it's a good idea to know which ones can and can't be combined before mixing.

Essential oils should not be confused with perfume or fragrance oils. Essential oils are extracted directly from real plants. That means the oil contains the true essence of the plant, including any therapeutic values the plant it was derived from has.

Perfume and fragrance oils are made from artificial aromas or fragrances, or they are made with artificial substances in addition to any natural compounds. Therefore, they are not derived from the plants themselves, nor do they have any therapeutic benefits. These are generally used just to give something a particular scent, such as in soap making or perfumes.

The chemical composition of essential oils and their aromas allows them to have physical and even psychological benefits on people. The most common ways to obtain these benefits are by inhaling the oil and applying it directly to the skin. The easiest way to inhale it is by using a diffuser. When applying it directly to the skin, it's generally diluted as the full concentrate oil can cause irritation to the skin.

Essential oils, either in pure form or blended, can have significant therapeutic benefits on people. There are many different uses for them, depending on the specific benefits of the particular oil. With over 300 different essentials, there is sure to be something for everyone.

Essential oils can also be used in massage. The essential oil is diluted with a carrier oil or massage oil and massage into the skin. This is a very relaxing method of externally absorbing essential oils.

AN OVERVIEW ABOUT DIFFERENT TYPES OF ESSENTIAL OILS & THEIR USES

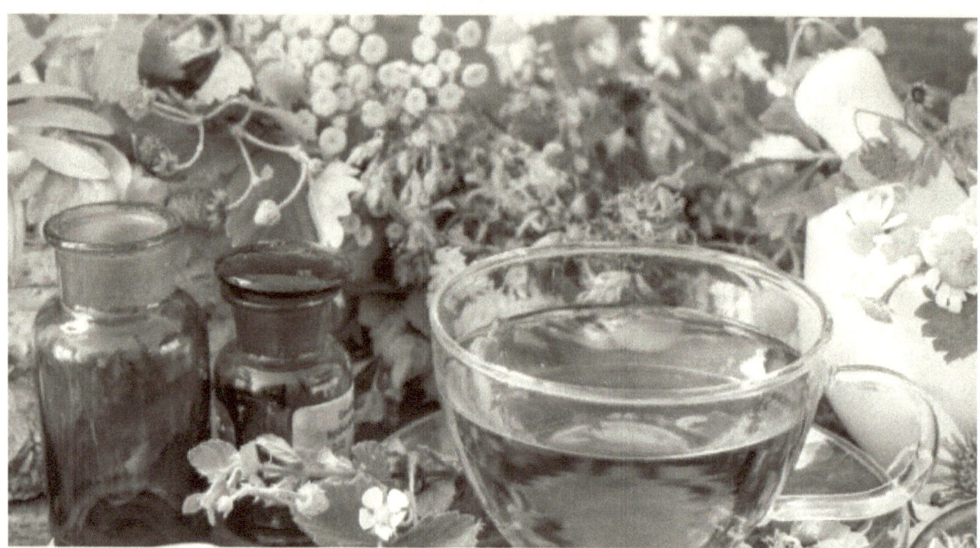

The essential oil is basically the oil that is extracted from the plant. There are various substances found in nature that contain miraculous healing properties. Owing to these properties, these products find tremendous use in several applications. The application area of the oils that are extracted from the plant includes aromatherapy, massage therapy, culinary applications, etc. The extraction of oil is a decade old process. It started with the invention of the distillation process. Since then, the extracted form of oil is being in use for various purposes including medicinal usage.

Some of the most popular forms of essential oils are discussed here.

Lavender Essential Oil - The most popular Essential Oil is Lavender; if you were only ever going to buy one Essential Oil then Lavender would be the one. It is used in all sections of The Essential 5. This amazing oil is one of the most useful of all essential oils. Lavender properties include antiseptic, relaxant, antitoxic, for burns, sedative, tonic, deodorant to name a few and blend well with most other oils. It is bridging oil for perfumes and is a very common known aroma.

Geranium Essential Oil - Geranium has a strong herbaceous aroma with similar notes to rose. This great all-round Essential oil has therapeutic properties as an astringent, antiseptic, anti-depressant, tonic, antibiotic, and as an anti-infectious agent. An aid against travel sickness assists with irritations associated with dermatitis, eczema, and psoriasis.

Lemon Essential Oil - Well known for its clean refreshing aroma it has high anti-bacterial properties. On skin and hair, it can be used for its cleansing effect, as well as for its antiseptic properties, and is refreshing and cooling. Lemon may assist with the ability to concentrate. The strong clean smell is commonly associated with cleanliness.

Chamomile Essential Oil - It is useful in the treatment of aches and pains in muscles and joints. Treatment of symptoms of PMS with Chamomile is also beneficial especially when the symptoms are related to stress. It has a long tradition in herbal medicine and the flowers were used in many cures including an herbal tea During World War Two. The strong aroma of chamomile is fruity and herbaceous and ideal for children and those with sensitive skin.

Tea Tree Essential Oil - Most of us have used or owned this oil at one stage. It is used in two sections and is best known as a very powerful immune stimulant. It can help to fight off infectious. Used as part of an inhalation it can help with colds, measles, sinusitis & viral infections. For skin & hair, Tea Tree has been used to combat acne, oily skin, head lice & dandruff.

Amla Oil - This is widely known as Emblica Officinalis. This is basically a fruit from which this oil is extracted. It contains various mineral & vitamin extracts. The oil extracted from this is rich in fatty acids, vitamin C, Polyphenols, Flavonoids, protein, carbohydrates, minerals, antioxidants, and water. This is very effective in providing nourishment to the hair. The application of this oil helps in providing essential nutrients to the scalp. It is very effective in providing complete nourishment to the hair. Its regular use helps in hair regrowth.

Cumin Oil - Scientifically, it is known as Cuminum Cyminum. The essential oil extracted from this is widely used for various medicated purposes. Its regular use helps in combating several diseases like diarrhea and cholera and various other bacteria-borne diseases. It can be used in the culinary application as it helps in improving the condition of the digestive system. In the case of gastric problems, it is very useful. It improves the functionality of the digestive system.

Betel Leaf Oil - This is extracted from the betel leaf. It is full of various essential ingredients that help in providing several health advantages. It is rich in various substances like calcium, vitamin, thiamine, and several other ingredients. It is very useful in combating several diseases like skin infection, gastric problems, oral infection, etc. Owing to its miraculous healing properties, it can also be used to counter muscle pain. It can easily remove stiffness of the muscle.

Carrot Seed Oil - The oil extracted from this vegetable is widely used for several purposes. It is helpful in providing nourishment to the skin. It is an excellent diet and helps in improving the blood level inside the body. Its intake helps in nourishing, tightening, and rejuvenating the skin. It can also alleviate pain due to menstruation.

ESSENTIAL OILS RECIPES

1. Coconut Oil Deodorant Recipe

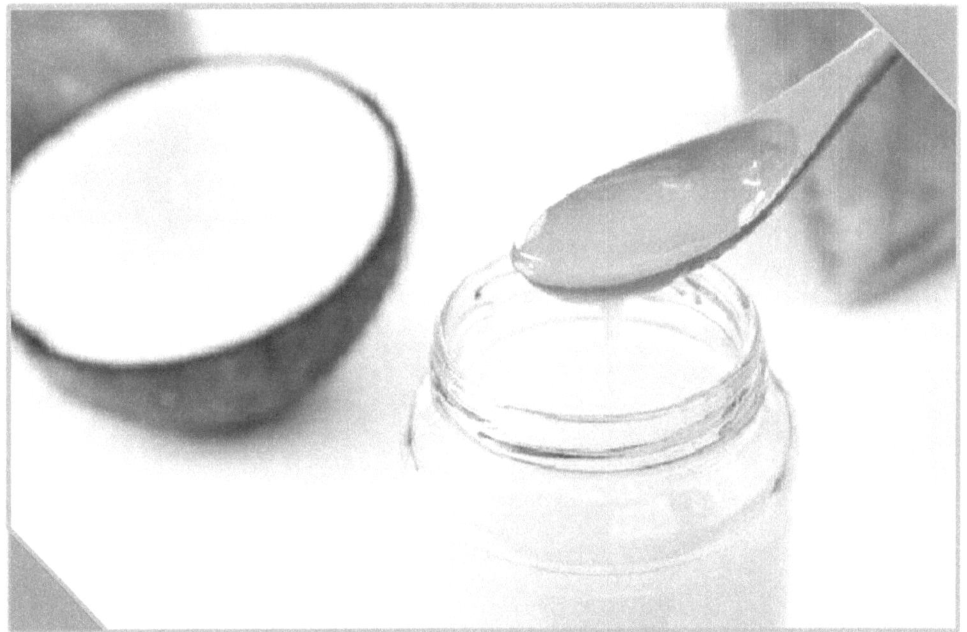

Ingredients

- 1/4 Cup of Baking Soda
- 1/4 Cup of Arrowroot Powder
- 4 Tablespoon Coconut Oil, Soft (room temperature)
- 1/4 tsp Essential Oils

Directions:

1. Mix all ingredients together until combined.
2. Store in an airtight container.
3. You can melt and pour the deodorant into empty deodorant containers.
4. If you have sensitive skin you will want to cut the baking soda down to 2 tablespoons and add 2 tablespoons of arrowroot powder.

2. Citrus Sugar Scrub Recipe

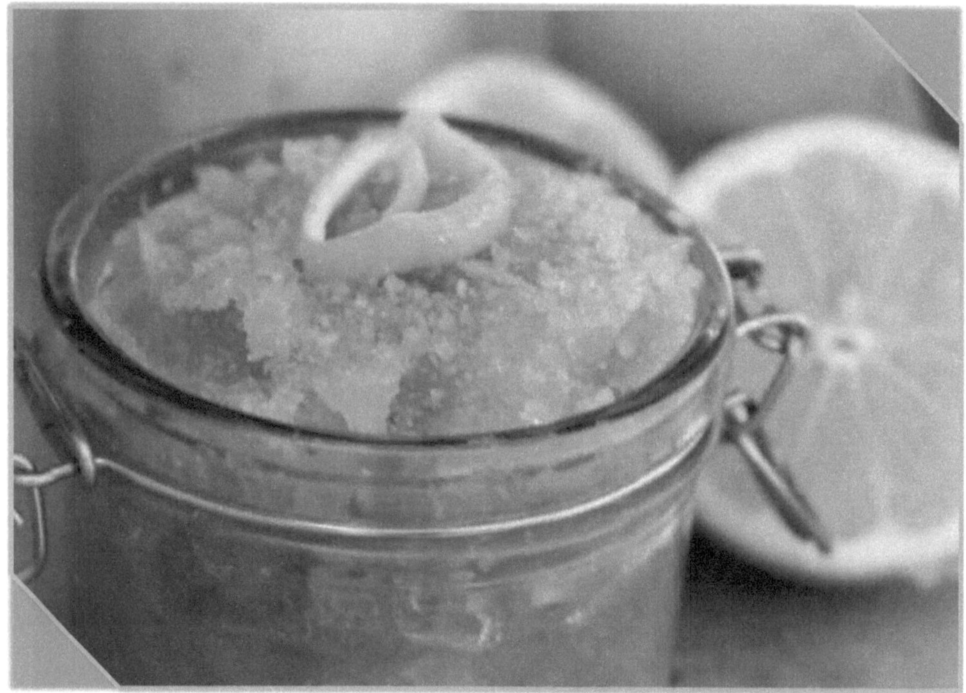

Ingredients

- 1/4 cup of coconut oil
- 1/4 cup olive oil
- 1 cup of cane sugar
- 20 drops lemon essential oil – substitute lime, grapefruit or orange oil if desired
- 2 tablespoons lemon zest (or limes/grapefruits/oranges)

Directions:

1. Melt the coconut oil until it has liquified
2. In a bowl mix together the olive oil, coconut oil, sugar, lemon oil, and zest
3. Mix until well combined and store in your favorite glass jar.

Use liberally on your body but avoid the face and eyes.

Note: Citrus oils can cause the sun's effect on the skin to be magnified, so use appropriate measures to protect skin from burning.

3. Diaper Rash Stick Recipe

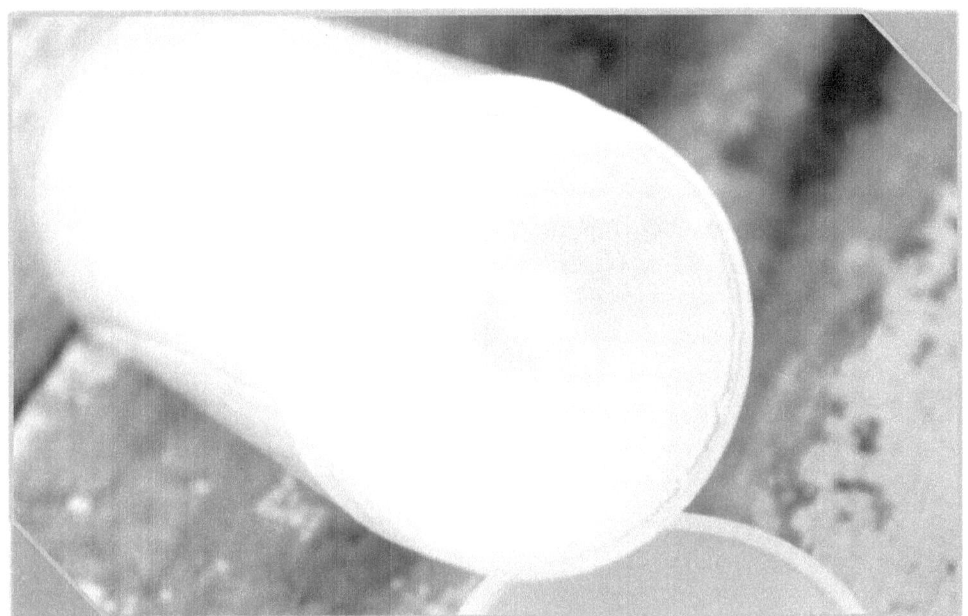

Ingredients

- 3 Tablespoons grated beeswax
- 1 Tablespoon shea butter
- 2 Tablespoons coconut oil
- 1 Tablespoon jojoba oil
- Essential oils (10 drops of Lavender and 10 drops tea tree oil)

Directions:

1. Fill a medium-sized pot halfway with water and turn on high to boil
2. Place beeswax in a mason jar
3. Place the jar in boiling water
4. Once the beeswax is melted add the shea butter, jojoba oil, and coconut oil
5. Allow melting completely
6. Turn the heat off and add the essential oils
7. Pour your liquid from the mason jar into an old deodorant container
8. Allow cooling.

4. All-Purpose Protective Essential Oil Blend Recipe

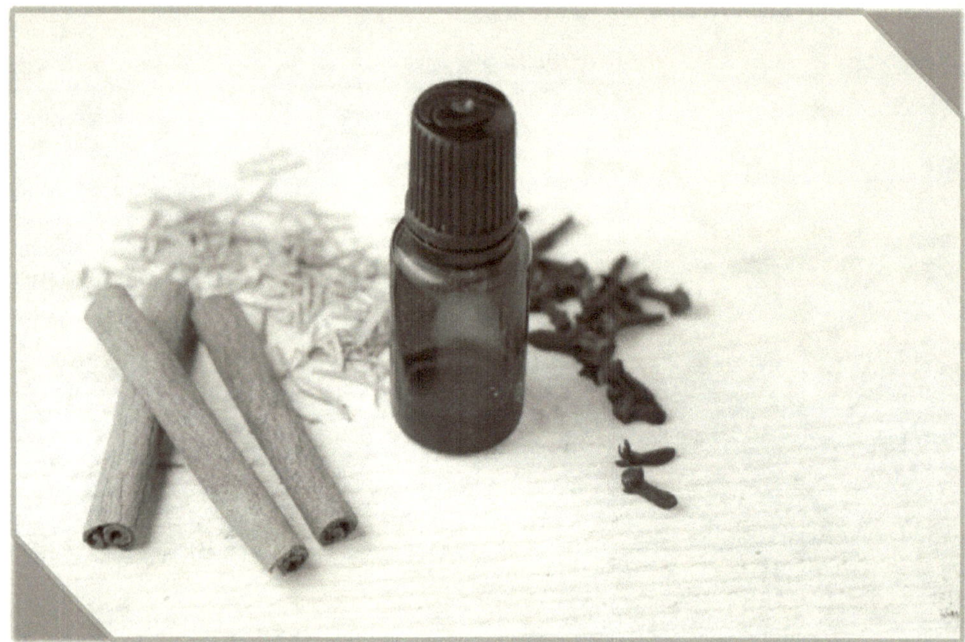

Ingredients

- 20 drops clove essential oil
- 18 drops lemon essential oil
- 10 drops cinnamon bark essential oil
- 8 drops eucalyptus essential oil
- 5 drops rosemary essential oil

Directions:

1. Combine all oils and store in a dark glass container.
2. This makes a fairly small amount, so feel free to double or triple the recipe.
3. To use this blend:
4. Use this blend in your essential oil diffuser to purify the air.
5. Mix this blend into your homemade cleaning products.
6. Dilute the blend, then rub it on the soles of your feet.

5. Homemade Vanilla Lemongrass Lip Balm Recipe

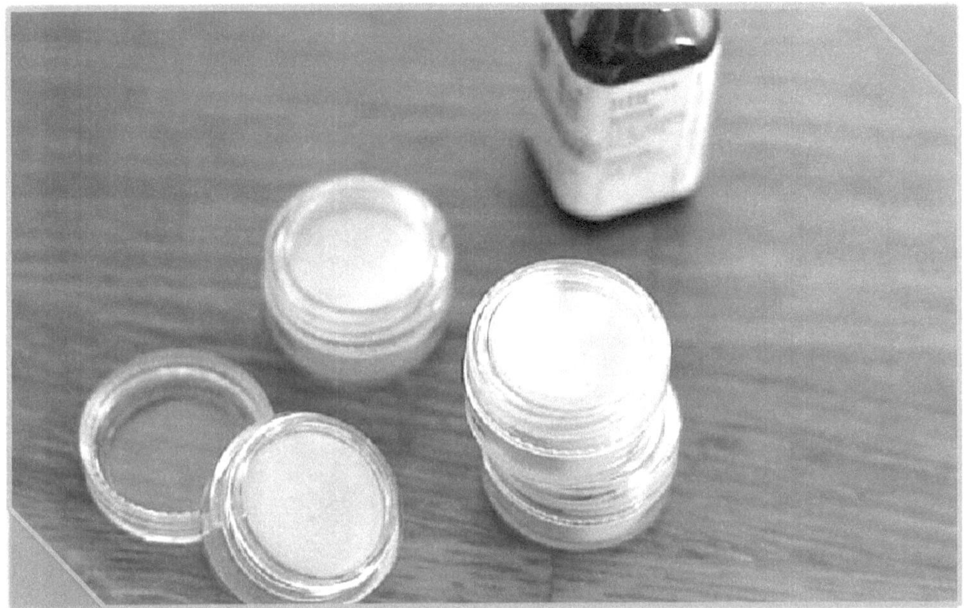

Ingredients

- 3 Tablespoons beeswax
- 3 Tablespoons coconut oil
- 2 Tablespoons shea butter
- 1/4 teaspoon raw honey
- 1/8 teaspoon vanilla extract
- 8–10 drops lemongrass essential oil
- Empty containers (you can buy these in a 10-pack)

Directions:

1. Combine the beeswax, coconut oil, shea butter, and honey in a small pot.
2. Melt the fats on very low heat and stir until they're combined.
3. Turn off the heat and mix in the vanilla and essential oil.
4. Pour into small containers. Some find that using a dropper or disposable pipette helps this process and creates less mess.

6. Peppermint Whipped Body Butter Recipe

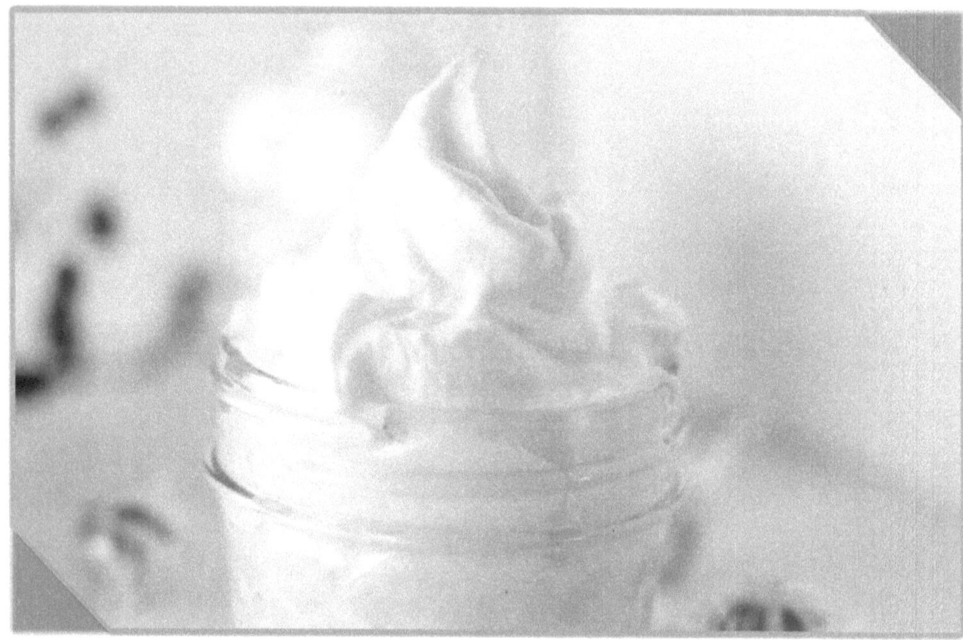

Ingredients

- 1/2 cup coconut oil
- 1/2 cup cocoa butter
- 1/2 cup shea butter
- 1/2 cup sweet almond oil
- 1 tsp vitamin E oil
- 2 – 4 drops peppermint essential oils

Directions:

1. Place coconut oil, cocoa butter, and shea butter in a medium-sized pot over low heat. Stir to combine until it melts completely. Remove from heat.
2. Thoroughly mix in the sweet almond, vitamin E, and peppermint oils.
3. Chill in your refrigerator for an hour or two. You want the mixture to firm up without getting too hard.
4. Once chilled, use a stand mixer (you can use your kitchen aid with the whip attachment) or hand mixer to mix until you get a decadent whipped consistency. Scoop into a jar or container.

7. Natural Homemade Vapor Rub Recipe

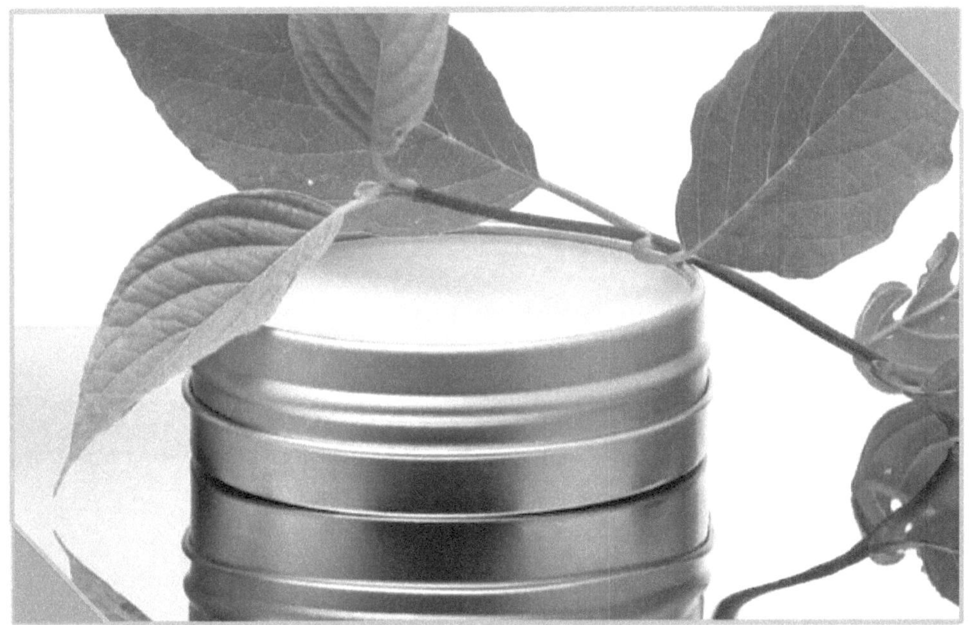

Ingredients

- 5 tbsp.extra virgin coconut oil
- 1 tbsp. evening primrose oil or other carrier oil such as olive oil or sweet almond oil
- 2 tablespoons beeswax
- 8 – 10 drops tea tree essential oil
- 15 – 20 drops eucalyptus globulus essential oil

Directions:

1. In a small pan, melt the coconut oil and evening primrose oil.
2. Add the beeswax, chopped up (or in granules) and stir until melted.
3. Add the essential oils and stir to combine.
4. Pour into a 4-oz. glass jar and allow to cool.

8. Homemade Deodorant for Sensitive Skin Recipe

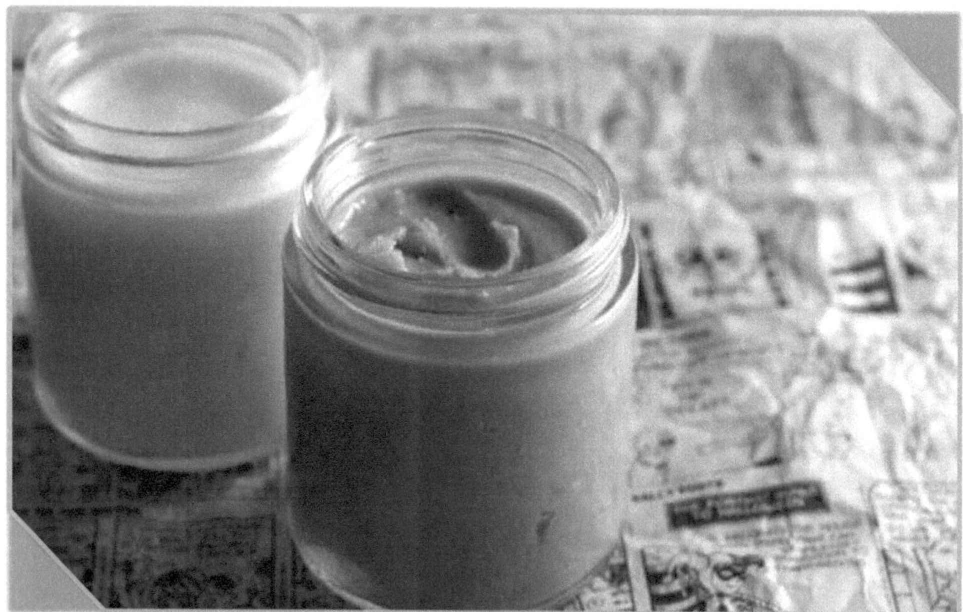

Ingredients

- 5 Tablespoons coconut oil
- 1 Tablespoon Baking soda
- 6 Tablespoons Arrowroot powder
- 2 Tablespoons Bentonite Clay
- 5 to 10 drops of the essential oil of your choice (you can use Lavender and Frankincense)

Directions:

1. Mix all of your ingredients together and store in a small jar in your medicine cabinet!
2. Your deodorant will be like a paste, so just scoop some out with your finger to apply.

9. Detox Bath Recipe

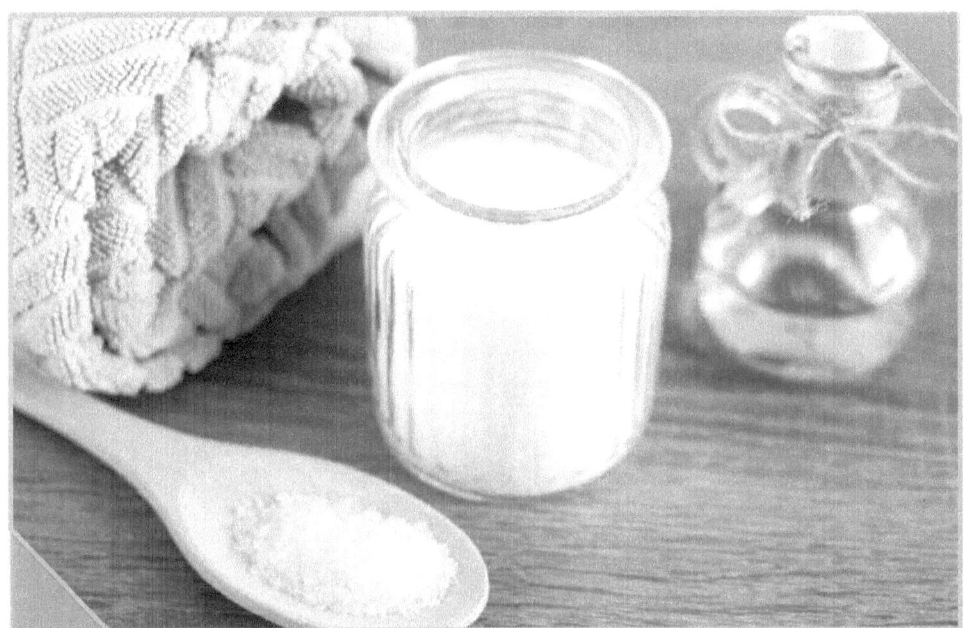

Ingredients

- Epsom Salt or Magnesium Flakes
- Hot tub of water
- Baking soda if the water is unfiltered
- High-Quality Essential Oils
- Coconut Oil or Olive Oil

Directions:

1. Add the Epsom Salt to a tub of hot water. Epsom Salt Dosage: for children under 60 lbs, add 1/2 cup to a standard bath. For children 60 lbs to 100 lbs, add 1 cup to a standard bath. For people, 100 lbs and up, add 2 cups or more to a standard bath.
2. Add the baking soda (optional). Adding baking soda to a detox bath helps to neutralize the chemicals in the water, especially chlorine.
3. **Baking Soda Dosage:** for children under 60 lbs, add 1/4th cup to a standard bath. For children 60 lbs to 100 lbs, add 1/2 cup to a standard bath. For people, 100 lbs and up, add 1 cup to a standard bath.

4. Add the coconut oil (or extra virgin olive oil). For a few reasons. One, it helps the essential oils to bind to the coconut oil and stick to my kid's skin which helps moisturize their skin. Two, it keeps the essential oils from sticking to the side of the tub. And lastly, it clings to skin even after you get out of the tub.
5. **Coconut Oil or Olive Oil Dosage**: For children under 60 lbs, add 1 tablespoon to a standard bath. For children 60 lbs to 100 lbs, add 2 tablespoons to a standard bath. For people, 100 lbs and up, add 3 tablespoons to a standard bath.
6. Add the Essential Oils.
7. **Essential Oil Dosage:** For children under 60 lbs and over 2 years old, add 4 drops to a standard bath. For children 60 lbs to 100 lbs, add 6 drops to a standard bath. For people 100 lbs and up, add 10 drops to a standard bath.

10. DIY Fertility Bath Recipe

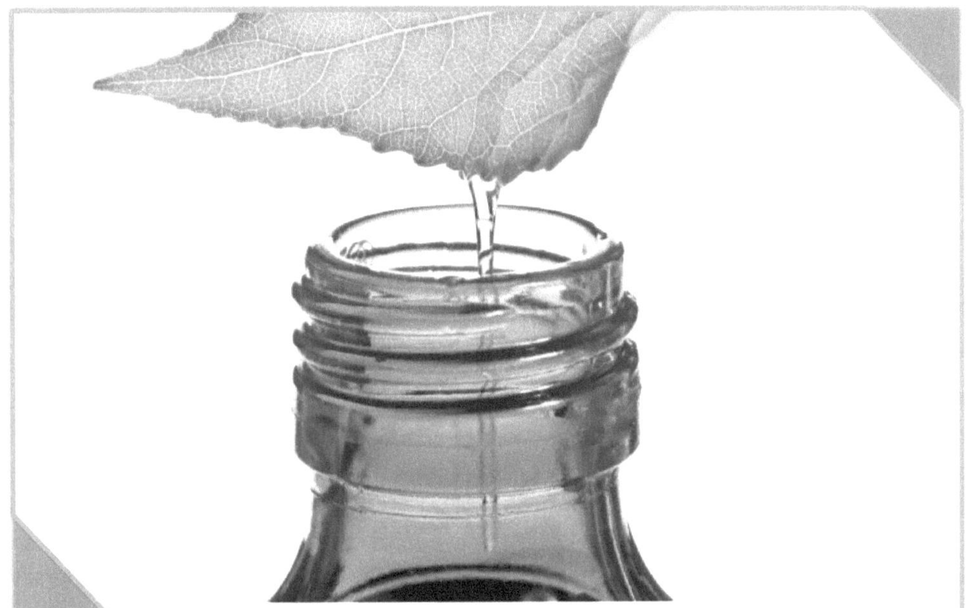

Ingredients

- 5 drops lavender essential oil
- 2 drops Joy essential oil blend
- 2 drops peppermint essential oil blend
- 1 cup epsom salts or sea salt
- 2 TBSP coconut oil

Replace 2 drops peppermint essential oil with

- 3 drops ROSE essential oil
- 2 drops Orange essential oil

Directions:

1. Run a warm bath, adding coconut oil and salts of your choice early on.
2. When the bath is full, turn off water and add essential oils drops on top of the water's surface.
3. Climb in and luxuriate! Enjoy this time for yourself and your body. Relax, have some quiet music on; maybe add a few candles to the room for soft lighting.

4. Be sure to hydrate before and after, as bathing in salts can make you a little bit thirsty!

CONCLUSION

Natural remedies basically consist of organic herbs and plant extracts known to cure diseases and common illnesses. Some of the popular herbal remedies today are those made from flowers, roots, tree barks, berries, and leaves. The big question is why do you have to choose these natural cures over pharmaceutical drugs?

Natural remedies and herbal medicines are known to treat as well as improve both mental and physical conditions of the body. They are excellent alternatives for prescription drugs and with no possible side effects afterward. Most of these natural cures can lower your blood pressure; treat diabetes, heart diseases, and even cancer.

Aside from being excellent in treating diseases, herbal medicines are also cheaper than pharmaceutical drugs. Why? Because pharmaceutical drugs need laboratory testing and manufacturing, which make these types of medicines even more expensive. On the other hand, natural cures are often from plants, fruits, and common household items you can easily find inside your home. These types of cure are not only convenient and accessible but also very potent making it very effective compared to other expensive drugs.

There are different types of natural medicines you can choose from; you might have already heard about Gingko Biloba, ginseng, slippery elm bark, uva ursi, raspberry leaf, comfrey, and the basic household items for natural treatment like honey, lemon, orange peel, etc. All these and many others are being used by different countries all over the world to give them both temporary relief and permanent treatment to their sickness. Natural treatment patients observed that with proper diet, healthy lifestyle, and regular exercise, they benefitted more from these natural cures, felt even better, and improved their overall health.

Of course, while all-natural treatments have no serious side effects to the body, it is also essential to speak with your doctor about your decision to take herbal remedies as your alternative medicines. If you are currently taking prescription drugs and you decided to combine natural medicines for treating your sickness, you might end up with serious side effects. Therefore, it is vital that you discuss these natural remedies with your physician before you take them.

www.ingramcontent.com/pod-product-compliance
Lightning Source LLC
Chambersburg PA
CBHW051232250726

48655CB00006B/2734